PARKINSON'S DISEASE: DIETARY CHANGES THAT WORK

Author: Lynne D M Noble

All rights reserved. No part of this publication may be reproduced, stored in a retrieval system or transmitted in any form or by any means, without prior permission in writing of the author Lynne D M Noble, or as expressly agreed by law, or under terms agreed with the appropriate reprographics right organisation.

You must not circulate this book in any other binding or cover and you must impose the same condition on any acquirer.

Independently published 2023

Table of Contents

Parkinson's disease - page 1

How to increase L-dopa - page 8

MAO-B inhibitors – page 11

Thiamine – page 18

Vitamin B6 – page 50

Magnesium – page 53

Parkinson's disease and cholesterol-page 56

Low protein diets – page 66

L-tryptophan – page 68

Methionine – page 72

L-tyrosine – page 76

D-phenylalanine – page 78

Octacosanol - page 85

Therapeutic cake and pate – page 88

Table showing the nutritional benefits of food items relevant to Parkinson's disease – page 92

Recipes to support Parkinson's Disease page 108

Appendix – phytochemicals for Parkinsonson, (129), Nrf2 Master Switch (133), Why protein matters for L-Dopa (138)

Glossary (140), vitamins and their key activators (143)

About the Author

Lynne Noble was born in 1953 in Huddersfield, West Yorkshire. From a very early age, Lynne showed an interest in nutrition and genetics avidly reading any books that she could get her hands on at the time.

Initially, Lynne studied orthopaedics but events led her to work with the elderly mentally infirm. Here, her interest in neurodegenerative disorders and pain syndromes developed.

Lynne undertook rigorous programmes of study, completing her Cert Ed., (FE) BSc (Hons) and Adv. Dip Education simultaneously before moving onto her M.Ed.

From there she took further demanding programmes in Human Nutrition, Pharmacology, Neuroscience, Genetics and Immunology. During this time, she was given many prestigious awards for her academic work. It was noted then that Lynne was not afraid of tackling difficult subjects.

She began her law degree but ill health prevented her from pursuing this. However, in this time, she moved from being a foster parent to adoptive parent.

She has been instrumental in setting up projects in the community for disadvantaged groups.

She is a member of the Guild of Health Writers.

Now retired, she lives with her husband in a historic Georgian riverside town in the West Midlands. She enjoys gardening, watching her husband bowling and researching.

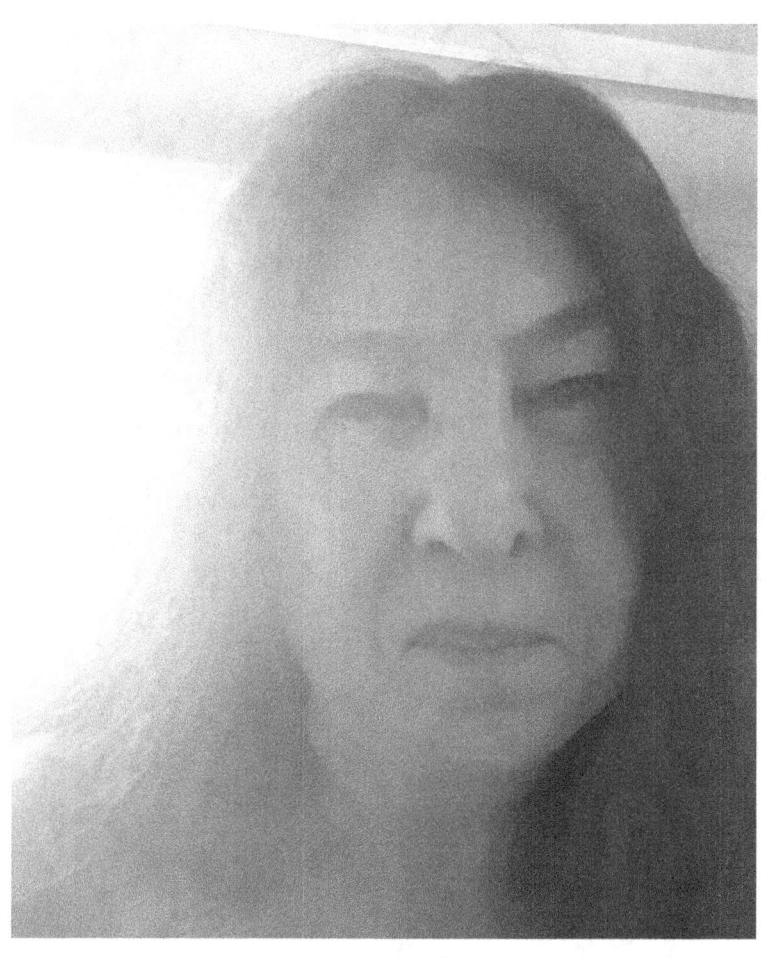

Author Lynne Noble, aged 67 years, at home

We do not 'get over' loss, we learn to live with it.

We do not forget those we have loved, we take them with us, talking of them often.

We can include their perspectives in our decisions & share the joy that they brought us

We can love because we were shown what love was

Copyright January 2022

Preface

There are plenty of books on Parkinson's disease. I had an interest in the condition but had not made a decision on whether to look at the reversal of or alleviation of symptoms until two events which happened quite closely together, occurred.

I had been contacted by a gentleman whose wife had suffered an encephalopathy which had resulted in the triad of symptoms which we recognise as being characteristic of Parkinson's disease. These are tremor, slow movement and shuffling gait. Of course, such symptoms were causing great consternation as the patient had also lost much of their speech and had limited walking ability.

Parkinson's disease tends to occur in the over 60's - although there is an early onset form – and becoming a carer, at that age, does not come without considerable difficulty.

The lady did not live near me. This hampered me somewhat as I like to see my patients. I can tell a great deal by looking at people. As it was the carer was an excellent communicator and provided such in-depth information that I was immediately able to formulate a nutritional response.

Less than three weeks later, the patient had regained their speech, the tremor had lifted, they were able to go walking with a companion. There was still some shuffling gait but I expect this to lift within the near future. Appetite was good and an interest in the world was beginning to return. Some anxiety was apparent but this did not surprise nor worry me. Healing in the central nervous system is normally slower than this, that I was witnessing, and I expect further recovery including less anxiety.

I cannot say for sure that this was Parkinson's disease – it had not been diagnosed as such – but the symptoms were similar and were amenable to nutritional treatment. In any case, Parkinson's like symptoms often develop after encephalitis.

More or less at the same time, a friend whom I love dearly *was* diagnosed with Parkinson's disease. I put aside the subject matter I was working on and began to pick up research I had begun a few years ago.

This is the result of that research and my notes, interactions and observations of many people with diverse neurodegenerative disorders including those with Parkinson's disease. I have learned a great deal from my time caring for those in residential settings as well as those I have met through life's journey.

Parkinson's disease

By the time that someone is showing symptoms of Parkinson's disease - and has been diagnosed with the condition - it is likely that between 60-80% of their brain will already have been affected. This seems quite shocking that a disease can silently damage part of a vital organ until most of it has been affected. However, there would have been some longstanding symptoms during that time such as constipation, depression, fatigue………. vague symptoms that are not attributable to anything specific like Parkinson's disease.

Later, apart from the triad of symptoms, which are: bradykinesia (slowness of movement) muscle stiffness and tremor, it is reported that

Depression, anxiety, psychosis, dementia, memory loss and sleep related issues also occur, among others.

 That part of the brain that is affected in Parkinson's disease is called the substantia nigra.

The damage leads to a decrease in a neurotransmitter called dopamine.

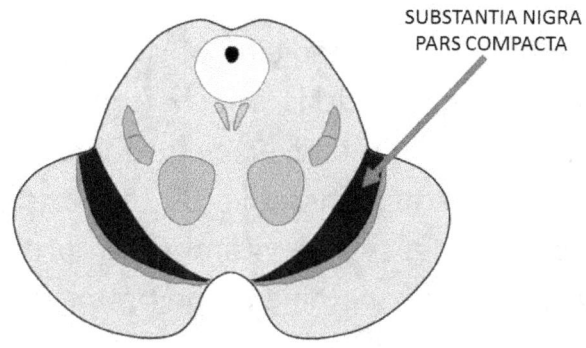

Dopamine is important in regulating body movement so the loss of this important chemical can cause all sorts of problems. The shuffling gait of Parkinson's is as a result of the loss of dopamine. The 'pill rolling' occurs as a loss of dopamine.

The shuffling gait can easily result in loss of balance, a fall and potentially fractures to compound the misery.

Levodopa is the medicine of choice. L-dopa is a class of medications which forms part of the CNS agents. It is converted into dopamine in the brain. It requires vitamin B6 (pyrioxidine) to do this. Deficiency of vitamin B6 prevents the synthesis of dopamine in the brain.

Vitamin B6 can raise GABA[1]. Glutamate decarboxylase and vitamin B6 converts the amino acid glutamine into GABA.

In addition, thiamine (vitamin B1) plays a beneficial role in Parkinson's disease by inducing dopamine release and improving symptoms[2]

The side effects of L-dopa are many. They include – but are not limited to-

Dizziness

---

[1] GABA is a brain chemical which helps improve pain levels, sleep and improves motor symptoms in those with Parkinson's disease.
[2] PMC 6493530

Diarrhoea

Appetite loss

Nightmares

Anxiety

Dry mouth

Constipation

Mouth and throat pain

Confusion

Altered taste

Poor recall

insomnia

headaches

weakness

Although these are general side effects, others are more serious and disabling. These include:

An irregular, fast and bounding heartbeat

Uncontrolled movements which may affect the face, neck, tongue and limbs

Increased sweating

Depression and suicidal thought

Swelling of tissues

Hallucinating

Chest pain

Numbness in the extremities

Urticaria

Hoarse voice

Problems swallowing and breathing

Nausea, vomiting, abdominal pain

Black or red blood in stools or vomit with coffee ground appearance

A fever

As L-dopa can cause patients to fall asleep suddenly, then it may not be safe to drive with the loss of independence that this can cause.

As if this wasn't enough, L-dopa can also cause strange and unwanted behaviours. People may suddenly develop sexual urges or urges to gamble that had not been part of their nature before. This can cause huge embarrassment for the patients and their families but it is not something that is easily controlled. The patient with Parkinson's disease should tell family members of these side effects so that should they occur, the warning of potential consequences may have given carers sufficient time to consider how to address these behaviours.

In this respect, joining a group for patients with Parkinson's disease may be helpful as there will be someone who has experienced similar and who may have a tried and tested solution.

There is an adjunctive medication which is often prescribed alongside L-Dopa. It is called Carbidopa. It is in a class of medications called decarboxylase inhibitors. It prevents L-dopa from being broken down before it reaches the brain. In effect it means that a lower dose of L-dopa can be given which can reduce the feelings of nausea and vomiting which accompany L-dopa. Nevertheless, Carbidopa had similar side effects to those mentioned for prescription L-dopa.

How to increase L-dopa

L-dopa can be increased naturally. Fava beans contain L-dopa.

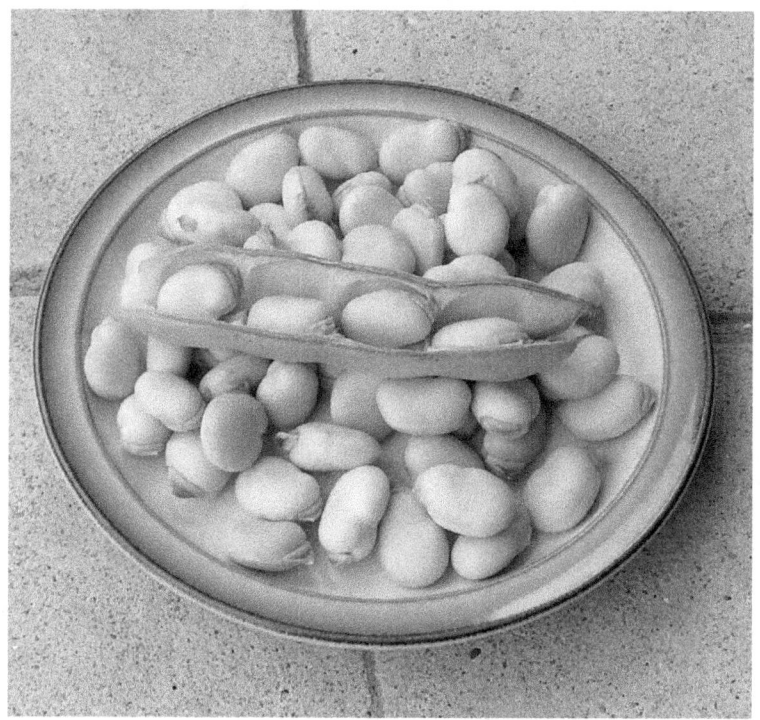

Fava beans, commonly called broad beans, contain L-dopa.

Fava beans contain enough L-dopa to have therapeutic value in Parkinson's disease. In fact, three ounces of fava beans (approximately half a cup) will contain in the region of 50-100mg of L-dopa. 100mg is the general dose of L-dopa given three times daily.

Young pods may contain even more L-dopa.

Mucuna seeds contain naturally occurring L-dopa. A powdered form of Mucuna seeds may be obtainable as a supplement. Follow the instructions on the packet.

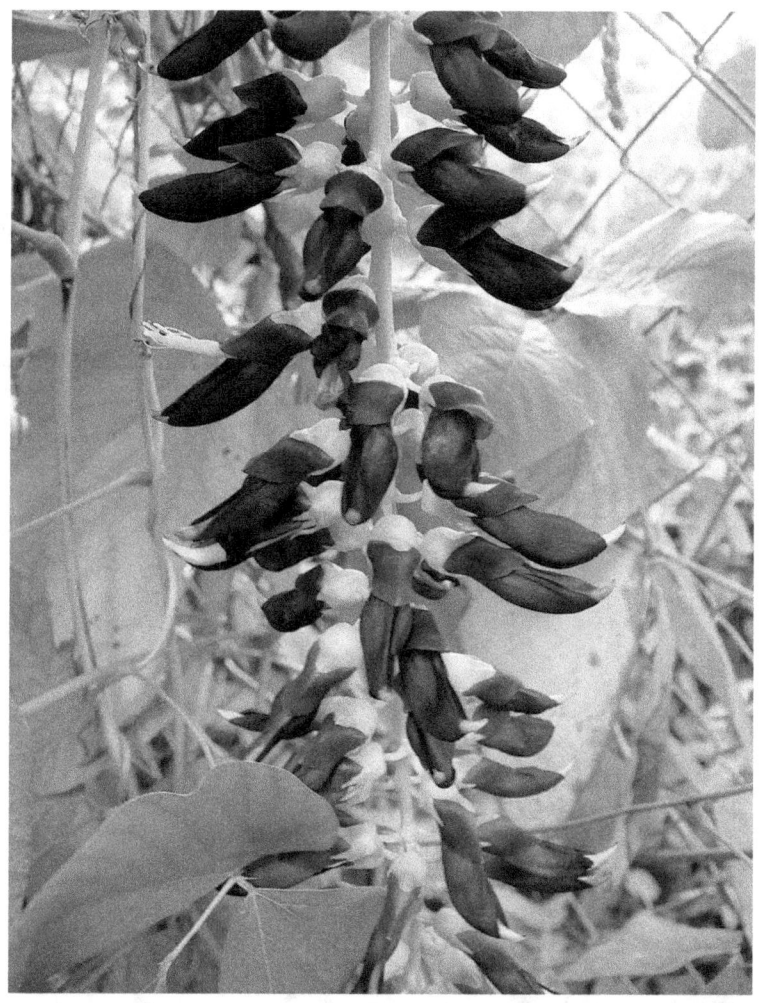

Mucuna seeds contain naturally occurring L-Dopa. This can be bought in supplemental form.

There are also foods which help the release of dopamine and these include:

Apples

Avocados

Beets

Dark chocolate

Coffee

Milk

Cheese

Dairy

Yogurt

Eggs

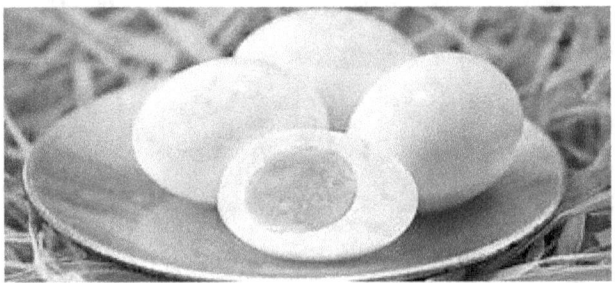

While some foods enhance the uptake of L-dopa, or the release of dopamine, it should be born in mind that iron supplements can bind with L-dopa and reduce the amount of medication that is absorbed by the patient.

The MAO- B inhibitors

The MAO-B inhibitors are an alternative to L-Dopa. They block the effects of The MAO-B which is an enzyme that destroys dopamine in the brain.

MAO-B is one of two isomers (the other being MAO-A) of a widely distributed mitochondrial enzyme. It is highly expressed in the brain, hepatic tissue and the gastrointestinal tract.

The isomers are differentiated by their preference for specific body tissue.

It is thought that the increase in MAO-B may be an age-related occurrence which impacts the central nervous system.

Knowing which foods contain The MAO-B inhibitors can also help us address Parkinson's disease. Fortunately, for us, there are many such foods and these include:

Kaempferel

Apigenin

Quercetin

Epicatechin

Hispidol

Luteolin

Piperine

Nutmeg

Liquorice

Fragrant ginger (kaempferel galangal)

Coffee

Curcumin

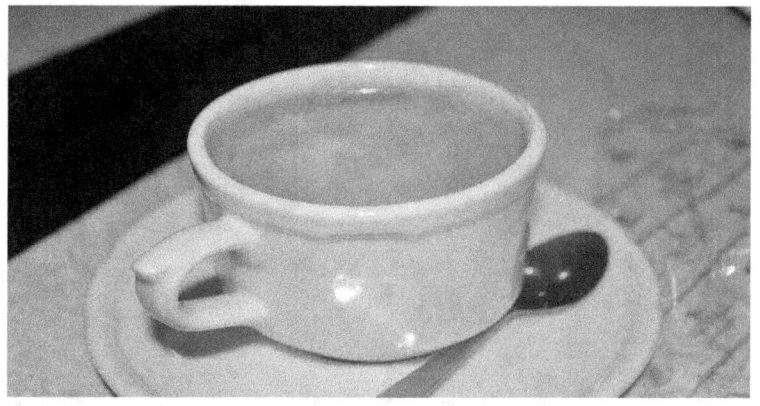

A cup of coffee is neuroprotective

Some of the above substances may sound strange but they are found in common foods and beverages that you will have in your kitchen cupboard that offer neuroprotection to those with Parkinson's Disease. Alternatively, they are easily sourced supplements:

For example:

Apigenin – easily sourced supplement also found in parsley and celery among other common fresh vegetables and herbs

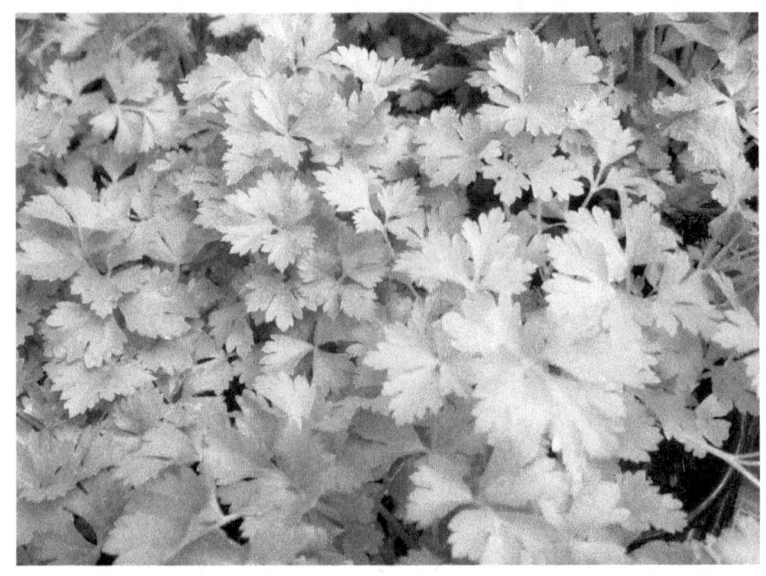

Parsley is an excellent source of apigenin

Quercetin – found in foods of the onion family such as leeks, all types of onion, garlic, ransoms, shallots

Epicatechin - cocoa, chocolate, red wine, tea

Hispidol - easily sourced supplement

Luteolin – apple skins, onions celery, peppers, carrots, broccoli and cabbage

Piperine – black pepper

Nutmeg – a common spice

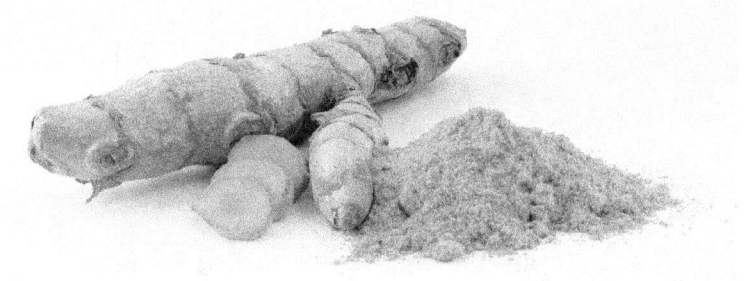

Curcumin an MAO-B inhibitor

Liquorice – proper liquorice not the black sweet type

Fragrant ginger (kaempferel galangal)

Coffee

Curcumin – the active ingredient in turmeric, the yellow substance used in curries. Suppresses MAO activity

The MAO inhibitors also increase thiamine (vitamin B1) in the form Thiamine pyrophosphate (TPP). The thiamine effect is so important to the health of the brain – as well as the rest of the body - that it deserves a chapter all to itself.

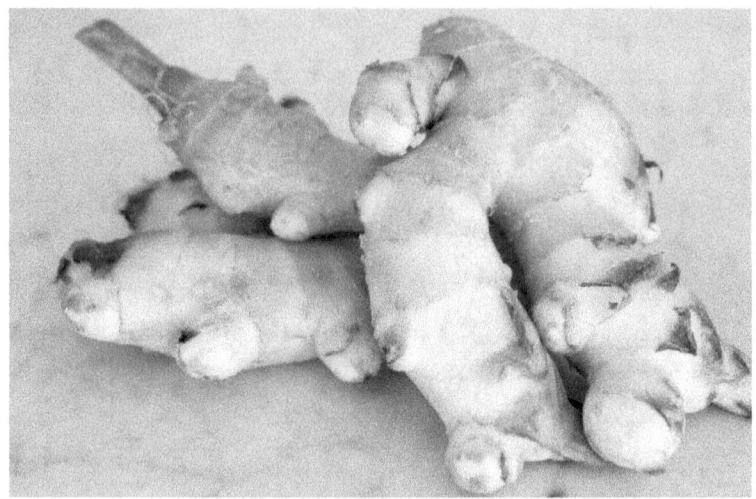

Ginger – a wonderful medicinal plant

Thiamine, wonder vitamin

Thiamine is known as vitamin B1 as it was the first of the B complex to be identified. It was identified by Drs B. C. P. Jansen and W. F. Donath in 1926 after being isolated from rice polishings.

It is supplied in supplements and in food fortification as a hydrochloride or nitrate

The Role of Thiamine Deficiency in neuro-degenerative disorders

Thiamine is a B vitamin (vitamin B1) and is a water soluble vitamin that plays a vital role in all cells. It acts as a cofactor for several important enzymes which are involved in the metabolism of glucose in addition to protein and fats. The importance of thiamine can be seen in the way it is involved in brain function as the brain depends on glucose as its preferred – and major form – of energy.

Absorption of thiamine occurs in the small intestine either actively or through passive diffusion. The intestinal enzyme phosphatase - through a process known as hydrolysis – breaks down the thiamine which is then absorbed in the small intestine. Once absorbed it enters the circulatory system to travel to key organs, involved in its storage, such as the kidney, heart, liver and brain.

There are many forms of thiamine but it is generally found in the body as thiamine diphosphate (TDP) which is also referred to as thiamine pyrophosphate (TPP).

It is perplexing to developed countries that deficiency diseases should exist in their communities. Therefore, the increasing numbers of individuals with thiamine deficiency occurring in all sections of society- but especially in the elderly - largely go unnoticed.

The importance of this vitamin for good brain health will be revealed during this chapter. Firstly, though, it would be helpful to find out why thiamine deficiency would exist in developed countries.

During the World Wars - and during times of depression - deficiency diseases were rife. Rickets, for example, was a well-known condition that was treated with 400 IU's of vitamin D. This was the minimum amount of this nutrient needed to keep rickets away. However, it was not sufficient to address the greater requirements of the immune system in the body.

As deficiency diseases were common, they were generally well recognised and responded to accordingly. Many children of the 1950's can recall being dosed with cod liver oil which was rich in vitamin D and vitamin A, malt for the B vitamins and rose hip syrup for vitamin C.

Children were encouraged to eat Marmite and peanut butter - both excellent sources of vitamin B complex - as they contained good amounts of these valuable nutrients. Liver and other types of offal were a regular part of the British diet due to their superior nutritional qualities.

Ovaltine, a barley malt drink invented by the chemist, Dr George Wander in Berne, Switzerland in 1865 contained impressive amounts of vitamin B6, niacin and thiamine. It was exported to the UK in 1909 and became a regular bedtime drink for all ages. Originally, it contained eggs as well as cocoa but the eggs were eventually taken out. Nevertheless, Ovaltine, as did other malted drinks, contributed to the overall nutritional requirements with regards to the B complex.

In addition, due to rationing, there was some calorie restriction which included carbohydrate restriction.

When rationing ceased, there was a move away from these highly nutritious foods. Milling techniques reduced the amount of available thiamine. The history of milling is itself worth studying in greater detail as it does impact on the availability of thiamine.

In 1940 due to the higher rate of extraction[3] of flour from the whole grain, it was recognised

---

[3] The extraction rate is the percentage by weight that is extracted from the whole grain to make flour. Whole wheat flour would

that the levels of thiamine were too low. An additional 200mg of thiamine was added to each 280lb sack of white flour.

In traditional milling, the loss of the nutritious whole grain is not as great as that in the contemporary milling techniques. Traditional milling techniques contain the whole grain which is ground and sifted very finely. Nevertheless, it contains the part of the grain which contains thiamine.

Modern milling processes are much more efficient so that during 70% extraction, the flour consists mainly of the endosperm. As a result, the level of nutrient is much poorer than milled flour with a similar extraction rate.

In 1942 there were grain shortages. A mandatory minimum extraction rate was set at 85%. As the highly nutritious wheat germ was kept – with only the course bran removed- thiamine was no longer added.

---

contain 100%. Ordinary brown flour about 80-85% and plain white flour around 71%.

There were various moves backwards and forwards with recommendations to add various nutrients to flour. The importance of thiamine was recognised during a review by the Advisory Panel on Bread and Flour of [4]The Committee on Medical Aspects of Food Policy (COMA) which continued to recommend that thiamine – in addition to calcium and iron – be added.

In 1988, the Bread and Flour regulations recommended that calcium - in the form of chalk - iron, thiamine and nicotinic acid, continued to be added even though a 1981 government report *Nutritional Aspects of Bread and Flour* stated that the original reason why these nutrients were added was no longer valid.

Nevertheless, subclinical, and often overt, thiamine deficiency abounds. How can this be so?

The bio availability of nutrients differs. Thiamine comes in different forms such as:

---

[4] https://www.sustainweb.org/realbread/flour_fortification/

Thiamine mononitrate

Thiamine hydrochloride

Benfotiamine

Benfotiamine is a fat soluble precursor to thiamine and needs to be converted to thiamine when, after conversion, its bioavailability is said to be superior to other forms of thiamine. In many cases it may be but sometimes the conversion mechanism falters in some people - with a genetic susceptibility that hinders this process - so that they do not benefit from what benfotiamine can offer to others. Further, those on low fat diets will not benefit from the fat soluble forms of thiamine. Additionally, benfotiamine does not appear to breach the blood brain barrier so will not have efficacy in neurodegenerative conditions.

Table showing the different forms of some common types of thiamine

Fat soluble thiamine derivatives	Water soluble thiamine derivative
Thiamine propyl disulphide	Thiamine mononitrate
Thiamine tetrahydrofurfuryl	Thiamine hydrochloride
Benfotiamine* [5] (does not breach the blood brain barrier)	Thiamine diphosphate
	Thiamine pyrophosphate[6]

---

[5] Benfotiamine is not a thiamine derivative but rather a precursor to thiamine

[6] Found in wheat, sunflower seeds and yeast

Unfortunately, additives are not always added with the best possible motives in mind. Prescribed forms of additives may not be the most bioavailable. They may be added because they do not alter the taste or texture of the flour too much rather than an addition which enhances the nutrient value. However, as they have been used to 'fortify' flour, the regulations have been complied with.

Bread making methods do contribute to the bioavailability of thiamine either positively or negatively, depending on the method.

Longer fermentation, such as that found in the making of sourdough appears to increase the bioavailability of thiamine.

Phytic acid may reduce the bio availability of thiamine – as it does with other nutrients – but milling, soaking and fermenting offset this to some extent.

The classical (yeast) bread making process is a relatively hard on thiamine content, leading to a 48% loss of thiamine in white bread.

The method of making bread is left to the manufacturer and is not regulated by the government.

From the above it can be seen that much of the original thiamine found in whole wheat is processed out during bread-making. The addition of thiamine to counteract this may not be in its most bio available form. Further, the bread making process, including baking, will result in further losses of this valuable vitamin.

Bread is part of our staple diet. We are led to believe that as it is fortified that it will be just as nutritionally sound as the original whole wheat but this is not true. Further, if the elderly have problems chewing they are more likely to prefer the softer white bread rather than the chewier wholemeal bread, thus depriving themselves of the nutrients that they need.

Further, just the act of eating carbohydrate – and bread has plenty of carbohydrate content – uses up copious amounts of thiamine. It would not be true to say that when all things have been taken into consideration that any addition of thiamine at the outset of the bread- making process would be adequate for our needs after eating it.

We need to look further into the sources of thiamine to see if adequate amounts can be obtained elsewhere.

We need to bear in mind that the Recommended Daily Intake of thiamine is 1.2mg but this is for normal healthy adults who are not involved in excessive exercise or have a diet or are on medications which prevent the absorption of thiamine. We shall look at this in more detail for this is not a definitive list by any means.

. Moreover, we would certainly need to increase this recommended amount of 1.2 mg for the elderly by at least 50% again for those not showing overt symptoms of thiamine deficiency and many times more than that for those showing some forms of neurodegeneration. This additional requirement is entirely reasonable when you consider that the ability to absorb nutrients decreases with age and that once a deficiency has occurred then therapeutic intervention only will correct this.

However, it should be noted, in case anyone is anxious about the administration of high doses of thiamine, that overconsumption of thiamine is unknown.

Unexpected benefits are seen in those with higher amounts in their diets or through supplementation.

Patients with Parkinson's Disease are recommended to take up to 4g daily and have shown symptom improvement with this amount.

Given the seriousness of any neurodegenerative disorder there is no reason why this recommendation should not be applied to the those with any form of dementia or degeneration affecting the nervous system.

Food sources of thiamine

The main animal sources of thiamine are pork. liver and fish. However, raw fish contains thiaminase which degrades thiamine. Therefore, raw shellfish or undercooked fish, is not to be recommended. Those with a liking for sushi may have to reconsider whether their intake is excessive or take additional thiamine supplementation to replace the lost thiamine.

Pork needs to be cooked well to cope with the increasing challenges of dentures. However, long slow cooking will destroy much of the thiamine that pork contains. Minced pork will need a shorter cooking time so may be preferable to a pork chop in terms of retaining thiamine. Lightly cooked liver is an excellent food for the elderly. All types of liver – chicken, beef, lamb's and pork liver have excellent amounts of thiamine with the latter mentioned having the most. I used to mince cooked liver and use it in a shepherd's pie.

Plant sources of thiamine are to be found in seeds, nuts, green peas, brown rice, beans and acorn squash. These are generally more acceptable forms of sources of thiamine but whether eating these on a daily basic can reach the RDI is debatable.

The RDA for thiamine was revised in 1998 by the Food and Nutrition Board of the Institute of Medicine. The reference value was based on preventing deficiency in healthy individuals. Every condition which manifests itself is a unique product of the convergence of many environmental factors. Thus we drink copious amounts of tea, coffee and alcohol all of which inhibit or degrade thiamine. We have a glass of wine as a night cap instead of malted milk. Alcohol is one of the worst offenders for degrading thiamine. It contains an enzyme, thiaminase, which breaks down thiamine so that it cannot be used. We shall look at the subject of thiaminase shortly. Moreover, we eat less peanut butter, liver and other organ meats all of which are excellent sources of thiamine and which were eaten regularly in the 1940's and 1950's.

Appetite reduces with age but whether this is due to sub optimum nutrition which can cause loss of appetite is not clear cut.

A table to set out the values is helpful.

Food item	Value	Food item	Value
Pork 3 ounce	0.4 mg	Beans 100mg	0.35mg
Liver 3 ounce	0.3 mg	Pumpkin seeds 1 cup	0.24 mg
Fish[7] 3 ounce	1.2mg (RDI reached)	Potato medium size	0.15mg
Green peas ½ cup	0.21mg	Inactive yeast (saccharomyces cerevisiae) 5g	2.4mg
Peanuts 3 ounce	0.45mg		
Almond 1 cup	0.30 mg		
Walnut 1 cup	0.45 mg		

---

[7] Raw fish such as shell fish and sushi will deplete thiamine rapidly due to the enzyme thiaminase in them.

There are lesser amounts in other food stuffs. They will add up to what is an optimum intake for any individual, depending on the storage and cooking methods used at the time.

Unfortunately, thiamine is depleted quite easily for a number of reasons. It is, in effect, a vulnerable vitamin. The most obvious reason is the presence of the enzyme thiaminase which is found in many foods, and beverages, that we incorporate into our diet on a daily basis.

It is to this that our attention will be turned to next.

Thiaminases

Any word that ends in 'ase' in the sciences is likely to be an enzyme. An enzyme helps speed up bio-chemical reactions in the body otherwise bodily processes such as digestion, breathing, even thinking would be far too slow.

Like the sloth everything we did would feel like hard work and take much longer.

Enzymes are great when they are in the right amount in the right place. They help speed metabolic processes up so that the body runs smoothly. However, inappropriately placed, or the synthesis of incorrect amounts of enzymes, will result in health problems.

As we age, we tend to produce fewer digestive enzymes. Why this is so, is a matter of debate and an important one at that. Digestive enzymes tend to be quite popular for those suffering from indigestion - and slow gut transit - in their later years. Could we assume from the popularity of these products at this stage of life, that the ageing process has something to do with this? As we shall see later, this is not so clear cut as it may first seem.

Individuals with chronic conditions may need to supplement with some enzymes in order to help their bodies, work correctly. However, enzymes are synthesised endogenously from nutrients like zinc and magnesium. If these are in short supply in the diet, then vital enzymes cannot be made in the quantities required for good health.

Thiaminase is an enzyme which breaks down thiamine into two molecular parts. At one time it was referred to as *aneurase*. It is referred to as an anti-nutrient when consumed as the degradation of thiamine by thiaminase renders it unable to be used in the body.

Thiaminase is found in many plants – most notably ferns – where it probably plays a part in plant protection. Sheep eating plants containing thiaminase will develop the condition polioencephalomalasia.[8]

Cattle can suffer from cerebrocorticolnecrosis and foxes eating raw fish which contain thiaminase often die from ataxic neuropathy.

Some bacillus and Clostridium have thiaminase in their cell. In a study the bacillus *Paenibacillus thiaminolytics* was originally isolated from the faeces of clinical patients suffering from thiamine deficiency. It was found that when

---

[8] **Polioencephalomalasia** – this is a relatively common disorder in sheep. It is often referred to as PEM or 'polio but PEM is a nutritional deficiency and not associated with the viral condition found in humans which is referred to as poliomyelitis

thiamine was infused into the colon of patients who were thiamine deficient, the added thiamine vanished. The bacillus which is a rod shaped form of bacteria, had destroyed the thiamine

The Clostridium botulinum serotype A2 is a strain which carries the thiaminase 1 gene. The breakdown of thiamine in this illness is distressing. Weakness and blurred vision, fatigue and problems with speaking are initial symptoms. Weakness of the limbs and chest muscle follow sometimes accompanied by vomiting, diarrhoea and abdominal swelling. Consciousness is retained throughout although the patient is helpless. Fever is not a symptom. Nevertheless, the above demonstrates the impact that lack of thiamine causes.

What we can take from the above is that a thiamine deficiency does impact the central nervous system and, in some cases, result in death.

Thiaminase is also found in tea – both black and green varieties – coffee, alcohol and raw fish.

The practice of consuming large quantities of shell fish or sushi washed down with a bottle of white wine, is guaranteed to cause a thiamine deficiency. It does not take long for such a deficiency to manifest itself in distressing symptoms.

Coffee is neuroprotective for those with Parkinson's disease but should be taken well away from the time when thiamine is administered.

Elderly in care homes are plied with cups of tea often with a biscuit or a small cake. A high carbohydrate diet depletes thiamine rapidly as does the thiaminase in the tea. Far better to offer malted milk as an alternative which would increase thiamine intake as well as other vital B vitamins.

Anti-thiamine compounds are found in some berries, mung beans, beets, Brussels sprouts and buckwheat seeds but, of course, the above provide beneficial nutrients and do not need to be dismissed from the diet unless they are eaten excessively. However, eating them 2 hours after supplementation with thiamine is wiser.

Thiamine is concerned with carbohydrate, fat and protein metabolism. It helps in the formation of the energy storage molecule ATP, in addition, it acts as a co-factor in enzymatic pathways responsible for energy production.

A co-factor is a non-proteinaceous substance which allows and increases a particular action.

Quite simply, if you eat or drink something with thiaminase in then the thiamine in whatever you eat at the same time, will be destroyed and thus unavailable for the body to use.

Thiaminases are denatured by heat but how high this heat needs to be and for how long is not known. Research is lacking in this.

Thiamine is also sensitive to heat. Prolonged heating splits the thiamine ring which destroys its activity. How long and high the heating has to be is unknown but it is more than likely that most of the thiamine added to bread will be destroyed during the baking process.

Chronic and severe forms of thiamine deficiency

As thiamine deficiency progresses, the condition known as beriberi manifests itself. During the 1800's, in Asia, beriberi was widespread. Christiaan Eijkman, a Dutch physician found that feeding whole rice, which contained thiamine, prevented beriberi. At that time, the Asians consumed only polished rice which was devoid of the thiamine found in the rice germ or bran.

There are a number of types of beriberi. The two most well-known ones are wet beriberi and dry beriberi. These affect the nervous system and the cardiovascular system, respectively. In addition, there is gastrointestinal beriberi and juvenile beriberi (whose symptoms are similar to childhood meningitis).

Alongside these four manifestations of beriberi, as dry beriberi advances, a condition known as Wernicke's Encephalopathy develops.

Wernicke's encephalopathy is a degenerative brain disorder caused by a deficiency of thiamine.

A deficiency of thiamine is generally attributable to alcohol abuse but - vomiting such as that found in prolonged morning sickness - the effects of chemotherapy, dietary deficiencies, anorexia nervosa or binge eating will almost certainly contribute to such a deficiency.

Wernicke's encephalopathy is characterised by damage to the brain's thalamus and hypothalamus. Although this is not the area that is damaged in Parkinson's disease, Wernicke's encephalopathy is long standing evidence that the brain is damaged by thiamine deficiency.

When many of the common neurodegenerative disorders are studied and research findings pooled, it appears that thiamine deficiency is the one factor that could account for the signs and symptoms of most of them.

We do know that patients with Parkinson's disease benefit from symptom relief from higher doses in the region of 4g. As we know that thiamine has no upper tolerable limit and is not contra-indicated with any other known medicine then it does not make sense not to try thiamine.

Just recently, a patient I was involved who had Parkinson's like symptoms – shuffling gait, loss of speech, severe fatigue, memory loss and pronounced tremor did, in less than a month of increasing thiamine up to 800mg daily, regain speech, lose their tremor, started participating in mile long walks and at the time of writing had begun to run. They were also taking on more and more tasks at home which had, at one time, been impossible for them. Not only is this hard on the patient but it is clearly very hard on the carer.

Perhaps the hardest task for any medical nutritionist is encouraging the patient or carer, to suspend their belief that conventional medicine is the only form of healing. In many cases it does not heal. Patients are attached for life to medications that produce horrendous side effects. The symptoms are relieved - in some cases - but the underlying disorder that caused the condition to manifest itself in the first place, rarely is.

The thiamine regime used in this case for a male in his mid-60's was:

Thiamine 300mg in divided doses throughout the day with 300mg of magnesium and a good B complex.

This was gradually increased to 900mg of thiamine daily with the magnesium dosage and B complex as for the 300mg dosage of thiamine.

Thiamine requires magnesium to activate it without which it is useless. People do not always take enough of either magnesium or thiamine in their diets and you cannot leave something this serious, to chance. Supplements really do help here.

All B vitamins work synergistically; they need each other to undertake a vital role so part of the thiamine regime is to include a good vitamin B complex.

Although there is a good amount of research to show the relationship between thiamine deficiency and Parkinson's disease, even if there wasn't robust research available, the rapid decline in symptoms, when thiamine is administered to people with Parkinson's disease, would be proof enough.

However, let's look at some of the research.

Onodera 1987 found that rats on a thiamine deficient diet developed aggression which was alleviated by the administration of dopamine.

Mizuno et al 1994 found a decreased activity of TPP enzymes in the neurons associated with Parkinson's disease.

Zaborsky et al in 2001 - mirroring my own experience with one of my patients - treated a number of patients who had acute neurological disorder with thiamine. The treatment was successful – and swift – given the severity of the symptoms.

This is just the tip of the iceberg of the many patients with Parkinson's disease who have benefitted from the administration of thiamine.

It is judicious to note that if the amount of thiamine given is too high then symptoms can worsen. Therefore, sensible incrementation of thiamine in a slow and watchful manner is the key concept. In this respect the carer and the patient can respond far more quickly to any changes than waiting for a hospital appointment. Both carers and patients tend to notice subtle and positive differences very quickly. These – as have been reported to me – are:

Looks brighter

Much more energy

Able to talk

Less tremor/no tremor

After being totally unmotivated for weeks, suddenly got up, after 3 days of thiamine, and started doing the housework

Walked for one whole mile – never thought this would ever be possible

Slept a whole solid 8 hours without once waking up which has not been possible for years

Went the whole night without getting up to go to the toilet

Some of the above happened within hours or 3 days of thiamine administration.

If thiamine deficiency is responsible for Parkinson's disease, then once the deficiency is corrected and the healing is as complete as it can be, then the next question to be considered is, 'Can thiamine be discontinued for good?'

There is lack of research on this. My own opinion on this is that it is likely that the factors that caused the damage in the first place will still be part of that environment or additionally, part of the vulnerability in that person's genetic makeup.

Supplements should always, once be healing has taken place, be reduced to the lowest amount that can be taken without a return of the symptoms but I believe that with neurodegenerative disorders that a minimum of 100mg thiamine with 300mg of magnesium and a good B complex should be part of that person's regime for the rest of their life.

Part of my reasoning for this is that a great deal of damage has already occurred in the substantia nigra before the manifestation of symptoms has occurred and it would be foolish to let one's guard down entirely and risk further damage to any part of the brain.

Thiamine rich foods do need to be included in the diet. Some of the best are:

Dried brewer's yeast

Yeast extract

Brown rice

Wheat germ

Nuts – especially pistachio's

Pork

Oat flakes

Liver - but bear in mind that liver contains plentiful supplies of iron which can bind with L-dopa and reduce the amount of medication that is absorbed into the system. In this respect a meal of lightly cooked liver would not be beneficial if served with broad beans as the iron in the liver would reduce any L-dopa in your system. Nevertheless, the B vitamins in lightly cooked liver are to be prized.

Those caring for loved ones need a crash course in medicinal nutrition which can be hard when all their physical and mental resources are taken up with caring for a seriously ill patient.

In addition, medications like Metformin (for diabetes) the proton pump inhibitors like Omeprazole and diuretics, among many others, inhibit or degrade thiamine leaving you deficient. Many of the above also degrade or inhibit the absorption of magnesium too.

We cannot, before we leave, forget the roles of vitamin B6 in the conversion of L-dopa to dopamine or the role of magnesium in the activation of thiamine, the wonder vitamin.

Lists of food sources for these two nutrients will be provided at the end of this book.

While supplements are often necessary in the initial treatment of a condition like Parkinson's disease, it is judicious to get into the habit of including the foods which address the condition so that when the supplements are reduced, the nutrients are still providing a supportive role.

Vitamin B6

Otherwise known as pyroxidone. It is a water soluble vitamin which is required for over 100 enzymatic reactions in the body. The main one is the conversion of L-Dopa to dopamine but it also enables the conversion of the amino acid known as 5-HTP to serotonin.

Pyroxidone has been known to counteract the effects of L-Dopa so supplementation is not recommended for this reason although foods containing vitamin B6 are vital for health and should not be avoided. In any case zinc supplementation may prevent this from occurring.

Other studies[9] have evidenced that supplementation of pyroxidone 10-100mg daily resulted in better bladder control, less ataxia, a decrease in tremor and rigidity.

The body cannot make vitamin B6 so it has to be taken in through food. Some conditions may

---

[9] Baker AB. Treatment of paralysis agitans with B6 j. Am Med, Assoc 116:2484, 1941

impair its absorption. These conditions include autoimmune disease, alcohol abuse, inflammatory bowel disease, decreased liver or kidney function or bariatric surgery. If this is the case, then increased supplementation is required and necessary.

NSAID's and oral contraceptives also deplete vitamin B6 rapidly.

Some deficiency symptoms include

Poor dream recall or nightmares

Low stomach acid leading to GERD.

Low energy

Anaemia

Migraines and headaches in general

Motion sickness

Water retention

High homocysteine levels (associated with inflammation)

Foods which contain vitamin B6

Beef

Tuna

 Beef liver and liver and organ meats in general

Greens

Walnuts

Eggs,

Salmon

Poultry

Sunflower seeds

Potatoes

Garlic

Bell peppers

Carrots

Dried brewer's yeast

Wheat bran

Yeast extract

Bananas

Brown rice

Main functions are:

Needed for the formation of the brain substances and nerve impulse transmitters,

Energy production

Anti-depressant

Anti-allergy

Blood formation

Magnesium

Half of magnesium is found in the bone and the rest is found in the organs, nerves and blood. It functions as a co-factor in many process especially energy production and cell replication.

It acts as a cofactor for vitamin B1 and B6.

It is involved in the repair and maintenance of cell and is a cofactor for hormones.

It is involved in nerve impulse transmission.

Deficiency is caused for similar reasons to vitamin B6 and may cause:

Weakness

Tiredness

Convulsions

Muscle cramps and tremors

Nystagmus (involuntary eye movements)

Unsteady gait

Irregular heartbeat

Palpitations

Hyperactivity

Low blood sugar

Painful swallowing

Good food sources are:

Beans

Nuts

Dried brewer's yeast

Brown rice

Dried peas

Wholemeal bread

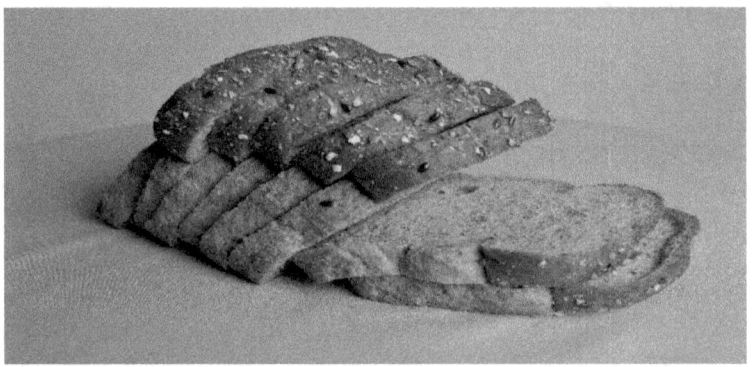

Sea foods

Dried fruits

Vegetables

Meat in general

Bananas

Green leafy vegetables

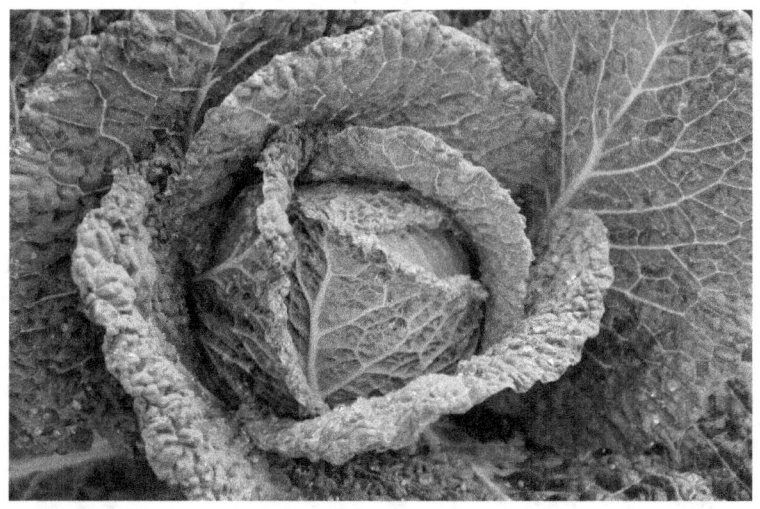

Cabbage is an excellent green leafy vegetable that contains vitamin B6. Be sure not to throw the cooking water out.

Parkinson's disease and cholesterol

Although statins have been popular for a number of decades, there is increasing evidence that lowering LDL cholesterol levels – allegedly the bad cholesterol - can have far a reaching and negative impact on a person's health. Firstly, though, we have to correct the myth that LDL actually refers to cholesterol. It doesn't.

Cholesterol is actually carried around on a raft. The raft is made from fat and protein hence the term high or low density lipoprotein.

The LDL carries cholesterol from the liver to where it is needed and drops it off. If it drops too much off then HDL raft simply comes along, picks it up and takes it back to the liver. You can see from this that there aren't two different types of cholesterol where one is bad and one is good.

When we look at cholesterol we see that it has a wide range of vital uses in the body apart from being required for the synthesis of every cell in the body. It:

Neutralises bacterial toxins which would otherwise spread through tissue destroying it.

It is required for the synthesis of every hormone in the human body

It is needed for the synthesis of vitamin D from the sun's rays

Reduces the risk of dying from a respiratory or gastrointestinal infection

It helps in the formation of memories and higher levels of LDL cholesterol are associated with good memory and longevity

It is required for the health of the brain and forms part of the myelin sheath which is the wrapping around the nerves.

This is by no means a definitive list.

Lower blood levels of total cholesterol including low levels of LDL cholesterol have now been found to be a risk factor for Parkinson's disease according to a South Korean study. Higher HDL levels were also good for the brain and were inversely associated with the risk of Parkinson's disease.

The study did not find any association between the level of triglycerides and the risk of Parkinson's disease.

The rise and fall of cholesterol levels should be of no concern. The liver makes what is needed and adjusts levels when required. We cannot do it any better and the prescribing of statins is not helpful and, in many cases detrimental to health.

Statins are a risk factor for neurodegeneration because they block the Mevalonate Pathway which makes Coenzyme Q10, a coenzyme which is necessary for the mitochondria to function correctly.

Mitochondria are the powerhouses of cells. Without mitochondria then cells will simply cease to function and die. While we synthesise plenty of Coenzyme Q10 when we are younger, we lose our ability to make this as we age. How this loss affects individuals will largely depend on genetic propensity. The point is though, that anything which disrupts the synthesis of a vital substance like Coenzyme Q10 is not good news. This is by no means the end of the disruption that statins can cause at this point on the Mevalonate Pathway, either.

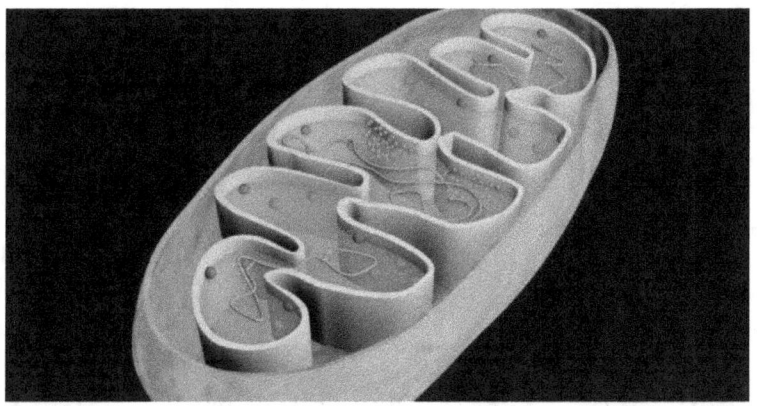

Mitochondria – powerhouse of the human cell

There is enough research to show that dysregulation of cholesterol metabolism is a risk factor for neurodegenerative process. This is not surprising since cholesterol is vital for the synthesis of myelin sheath as well as the cell membranes I mentioned earlier. Indeed, the brain contains more cholesterol than anywhere else in the body which shows the importance of this substance.

A study found that mice with cholesterol synthesis deficiency develop tremor and ataxia.[10]

---

[10] https://www.nature.com/articles/s41598-022-25180-8#ref-CR22

Abnormal serum cholesterol levels are a risk factor for other neurodegenerative disorders like amyotrophic lateral sclerosis and Huntington's disease[11]

However, the connection between abnormal serum levels and cholesterol found in the brain is not so straightforward. Lipoprotein rafts do not readily cross the blood brain barrier so any connection is an indirect one.

Abnormal cholesterol levels do not generally occur unless there is intervention through medication.

Cholesterol levels were lowered in the 1950's without any evidence that they caused cardiovascular disease. Nevertheless, the alleged association continues to be aired – and very successfully it appears too. The original levels of cholesterol have never been returned to. The impossibly low levels of cholesterol mean that most of the over 55's are mass

---

[11] https://www.nature.com/articles/s41598-022-25180-8#ref-CR24

medicated with something that is now known to be harmful to the central nervous system.

There is really no need to increase your cholesterol intake nor try to reduce levels through special – and often expensive – specially made plant based drinks or yogurts. The liver is a complex and wonderful organ and it does know exactly how much cholesterol it needs to make on a minute by minute basis.

Bear in mind that Professor John Yudkin found that cardiovascular disease was related to sugar not cholesterol and it is unwise to lower a vital substance in the body, artificially.

If anyone is still concerned about their own unique cholesterol levels, then the administration of one gram of vitamin C will correct any underlying abnormality. Those who are smokers or have malabsorption problems, are on diuretics or under stress may have to double this. Vitamin C is used up very quickly at times of illness or stressful events.

Plaque accumulates in arteries when some of the B complex are deficient particularly pyroxidone (vitamin B6) and folate (vitamin B9). In addition, vitamin K2 is needed to clear out arteries and keep them flexible.

Lists of good sources of the vitamin B9 and vitamin K2 will be given below.

Sources of folate (synthetic form is folic acid)

Folic acid was found to be a growth factor for bacteria in 1940

Food sources are:

Dried brewer's yeast

Soya flour

Wheat germ and wheat bran

Nuts

Pigs liver

Green leafy vegetables

Wholegrains

Pig's kidney

Pulses (beans)

Citrus fruits

Eggs

Brown rice

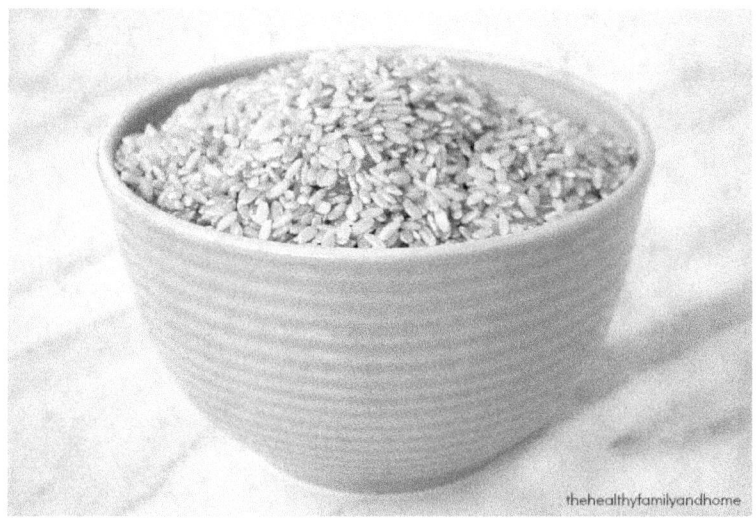

Brown rice contains folic acid

Food sources of vitamin K2

Vitamin K2 is synthesised in the intestine by gut bacteria so does not need to be supplemented. Nevertheless, **fermented** foods such as cheese, yogurt, kimchi, kefir also supply vitamin K2.

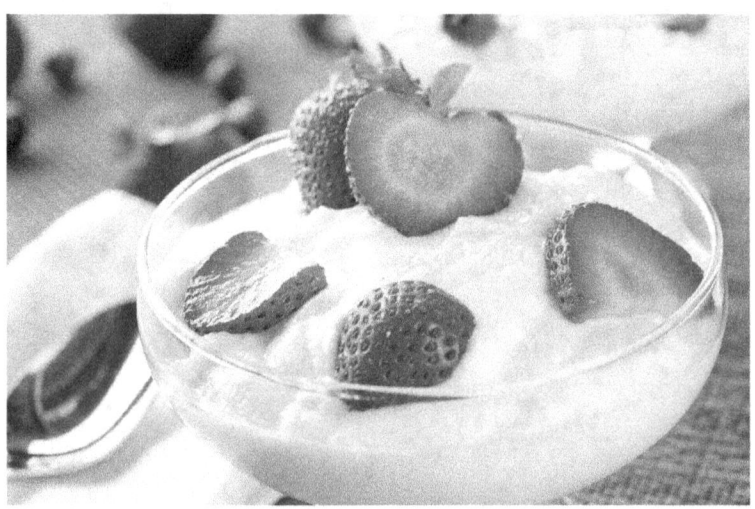

Yogurt is an excellent source of vitamin k2

Low protein diets and Parkinson's disease

A low protein diet may control the motor fluctuations seen in patients who receive L-dopa and carbidopa.

In one study 11 patients were placed on a very low protein diet. Sensitivity to L-dopa was found to be increased and this lessened movement fluctuation. This meant that a reduction in L-dopa could be implemented and the adjuvants stopped completely.

Vitamin C

Supplementation of vitamin C has been found to counteract the negative side effects of L-dopa.

In an experimental double blind case study, a 62-year-old male had stopped L-dopa because of the side effects which include nausea and salivating.

L-dopa was started again but this time with supplementation of vitamin C. Within a month the participant was salivating less, playing the piano, was able to move his head better, speech and handwriting improved.

To see whether these improvements were due to other than the vitamin C, the vitamin C was withdrawn and something else substituted. Every time the symptoms returned but once the vitamin C was introduced again, the symptoms lessened again. This was undertaken as a double blind trial. [12]

Vitamin C is, of course, found in fresh fruit and vegetables but it may be difficult to obtain as much as would be required to see the changes mentioned in the study.

Supplementing with ascorbic acid at 2-3g daily in divided doses would be necessary. Sometimes ascorbic acid can be a little hard on the stomach although I have never found it so, if this is the case there is a non-acidic form although it does tend to be more expensive.

---

[12] Sacks W. Lancet March 1975

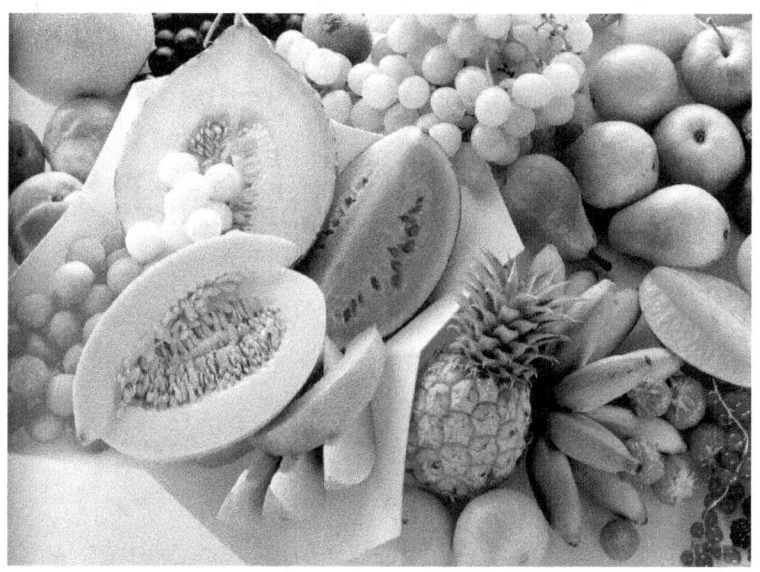

fruit – full of vitamin C

L-tryptophan

L-tryptophan is a large amino acid which has a diverse range of benefits. It is a precursor to serotonin, the happy hormone. It is an effective analgesic and it shortens sleep latency.

Supplementation may be beneficial for patients on L-dopa because L-dopa and L-tryptophan compete with each other and L-dopa wins. Malabsorption of L-tryptophan occurs and may result in depression for the patient with Parkinson's disease.

In one experimental study, mental disturbance was observed in patients with low levels of tryptophan. When oral tryptophan was started, mood improved.

Tryptophan is taken in 500mg doses up to three times daily.

As it is such a large molecule and competes with smaller amino acids, it is better taken with half a biscuit which will aid its transport through the blood brain barrier.

Tryptophan is found in a wide range of foods including:

Turkey breast

Poultry in general

Tuna

Beans

lentils

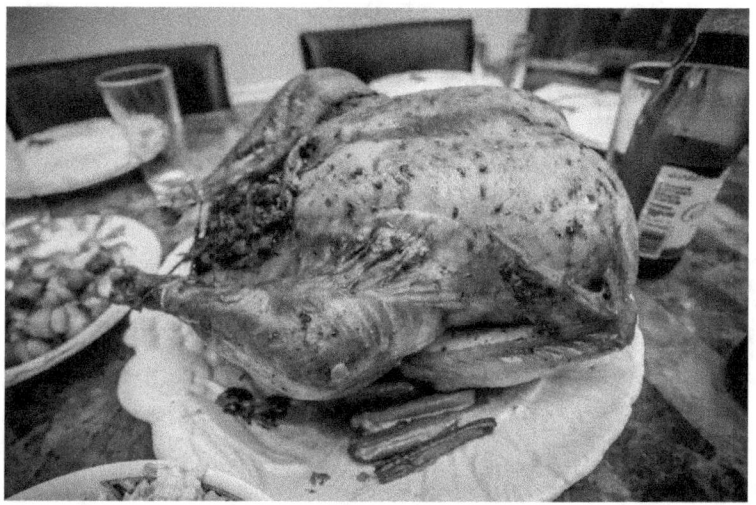

Poultry is a good source of tryptophan

Leucine

Leucine is an amino acid that may help some patients with Parkinson's disease when it is supplemented. 5% of patients with Parkinson's have olivopontocerebellar atrophy which is generally due to a deficiency of the enzyme glutamate dehydrogenase which can cause glutamic acid toxicity.

In an experimental study[13], 50% of 6 patients improved over 6 months when they received leucine at 10gms daily. The disease remained stable for 1/3 of them.

Leucine is an essential amino acid which means that it must be obtained from diet. It is known as a branched chain amino acid. They tend to be deficient in the amino acid profiles of chronically sick individuals including those with Parkinson's disease.

Salmon

Chickpeas

Brown rice

Eggs

Soybeans

---

[13] Duvoisin RC, neurology, chairman, U. of Medicine and Dentistry of New Jersey –Rutgers Medical School – quoted in Med. World News November 8, 1982

Beef

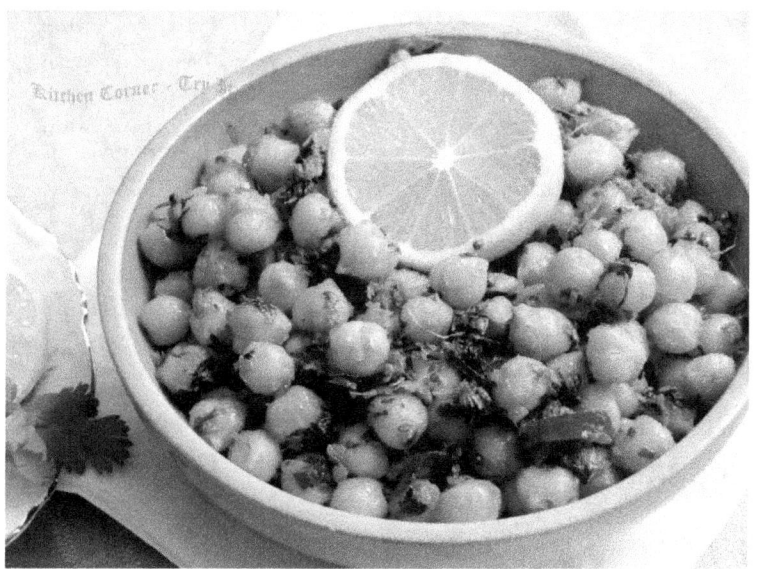

Chickpeas are a good source of the amino acid leucine

Methionine

Methionine is an essential amino acid containing sulphur. It is a powerful antioxidant providing protection against free radical damage to tissues. It needs the assistance of vitamin B6 in order to be able to function properly.

It is assists gall bladder function by being used in the synthesis of bile salts.

It helps produce choline and adrenaline, lecithin and the important vitamin for brain health, vitamin B12.

It is the precursor of many other amino acids – cysteine, cysteine and taurine.

It chelates many of the heavy metals and removes them from the body.

It helps remove excess histamine from the body and so it useful in allergic conditions.

It prevents the build-up of fats in the liver

Finally, it is essential for making selenium bioavailable.

In regards to Parkinson's disease it may help at doses of 1-5g given daily for two months.

A deficiency leads to hair loss, non-alcoholic fatty liver disease, anaemia and atherosclerosis. These other symptoms of methionine deficiency are useful to know so that they can be addressed before they cause a problem.

Sources of methionine

The animal sources of methionine include: salmon

Shrimp

Beef

Lamb

Tuna – tuna is probably the best source as a four ounce serving contains over 100% of the recommended daily intake.

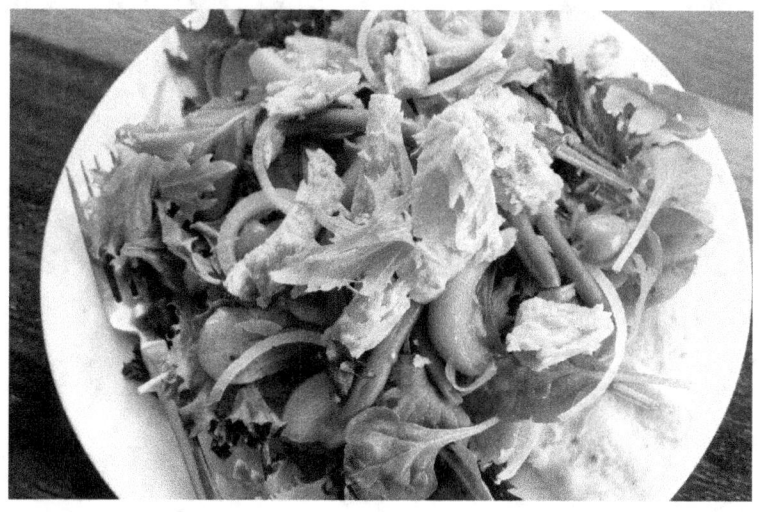

Tuna contains admirable amounts of methionine

Plant based sources include brazil nuts

wheat germ

spirulina

tofu

beans

lentils

soybeans

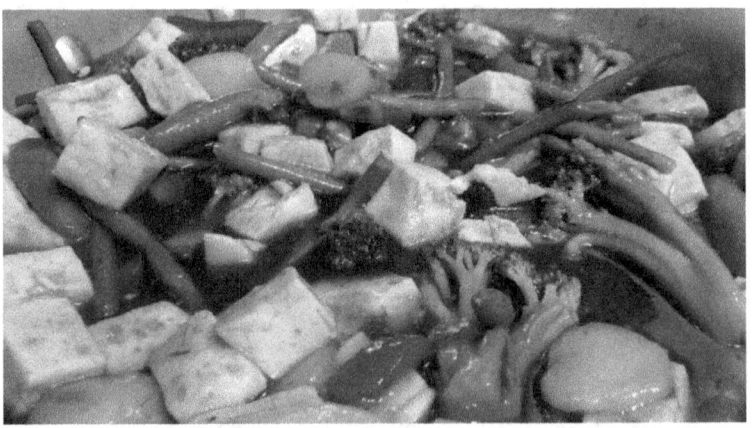

Tofu is a vegan source of methionine

L-tyrosine

L-tyrosine is an amino acid that is derived from phenylalanine. It is a precursor of the thyroid hormones and of dopa, dopamine, noradrenaline and adrenaline.

It increases dopamine turnover to enhance its transmission.

It is vital in aiding normal brain function and supplies neurotransmitters where abnormal brain function occurs. This would, of course, include those in short supply with those with Parkinson's disease.

Although it is well known for treating depression in those not amenable to tryptophan, it is useful for treating Parkinson's disease. However, the smaller doses appear to be more effective in raising neurotransmitter levels.

In an experimental study, supplementation with L-tyrosine 100mg/kg/daily increased cerebral spinal fluid (CSF) levels of tyrosine and homovanillic acid. Homovanillic acid is the major dopamine metabolite.

In this study, 23 patients were pre-treated with probenecid which is a renal tubular blocking agent. The increased CSF levels suggested that supplementation with L-tyrosine can enhance dopamine turnover.

It would be unusual to find a tyrosine deficiency unless there is a reduced intake of the animal proteins which are the major sources of D-phenylalanine.

Thus mainly plant based diets or poor eating habits will have the potential to reduce the neurotransmitters required to avoid Parkinsonian symptoms.

Good sources of tyrosine include: chicken, pumpkin seeds, sesame seeds, lima beans, cottage cheese. turkey, fish, peanuts, avocados, almonds, bananas, milk, cheese and yogurt although this is not a definitive list

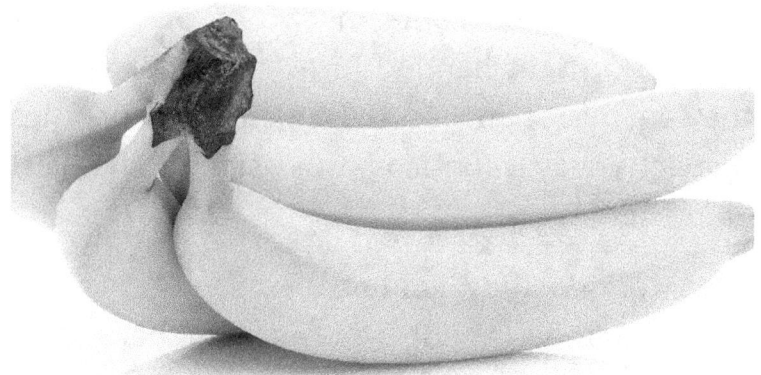

Bananas are a great source of L-tyrosine

Supplementation of L-tyrosine is normally administered at 100mg per kg of body weight.

D-phenylalanine

Supplementation may be helpful for those with Parkinson's disease.

D-phenylalanine has in one experimental study [14]found to made significant improvements in rigidity, walking, gait, speech difficulties and depression.

---

[14] Heller B et al, Therapeutic action of D-phenylalanine in Parkinson's disease Arnheim-Forsch 26:577-79, 1976

The amino acids come in two forms – a left handed or right handed form. In other words, they are mirror images of each but in every other respect they contain the same chemical elements.

Even though they contain the same chemical elements they cannot be used interchangeably just as a glove for the right hand cannot be used by the left.

The body is generally constructed from the L form and nature is constructed from the D forms. Although the amino acids we use tend to be the L form, sometimes the D form comes in useful and does have therapeutic value. The D form of phenylalanine has value for treating pain.

However, when we see an amino acid without a handle to it such as tyrosine then we can safely assume that it is the 'L' form. Forms which contain both D and L form will be name as such. For example, you may see D-L phenylalanine which will contain both forms.

The essential amino acid for the adult body are:

L-tryptophan

L-isoleucine

L-lysine

L-threonine

L-leucine

L-methionine

L-phenylalanine

L-valine

We can now assume that if an amino acid is named, that it is the 'L' form. If a 'D' form or a 'DL' form it will be prescribed as such.

In an experimental study of the benefits of D-phenylalanine and the aforementioned benefits. Fifteen patients received DPA 1-250mg twice daily. After 4 weeks, repeat neurological examinations revealed significant improvements in the aforementioned symptoms.

Now bear in mind that all the patients improved. With some supplements, not all patients will improve because they may lack a deficiency elsewhere. For example, take the hypothetical case of a patient with Parkinson's who eats enough broad beans to provide all the L-dopa to treat the condition but does not address a pyroxidone deficiency. Without vitamin B6 the L-dopa in the beans cannot be transformed into dopamine.

Whenever we investigate any condition we have to be mindful of the numerous steps involved and required to keep it healthy and working.

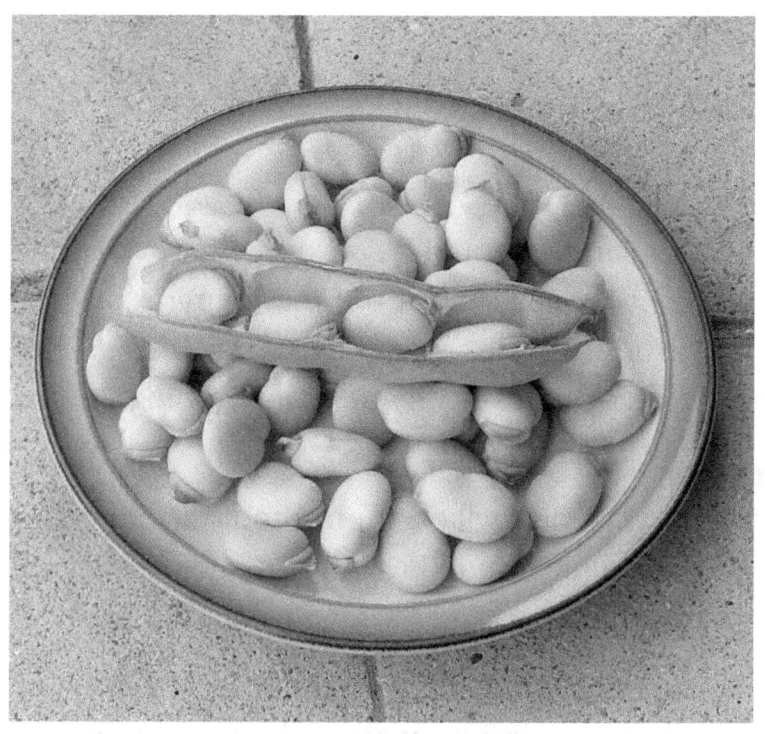

Broad beans and vitamin B6 are needed to provide L-dopa and convert it to the neurotransmitter, dopamine.

A phenylalanine deficiency may start in childhood – as do many deficiencies – it leads to a tyrosine deficiency and mental retardation as well as a melanin deficiency.

When a melanin deficiency occurs then eczema is more likely to occur. In adults a deficiency of phenylalanine results in:

Weight gain

Circulatory problems

Emotional disorders

Phenylalanine should never be taken by anyone currently taking any of the monoamine oxidase inhibitor drugs commonly known as MAO's. They should not be taken by anyone with high blood pressure.

Those with phenylketonuria should avoid and it is contraindicated in lactating or pregnant women.

If you are trying to avoid phenylalanine, then be aware that soda pop tends to be a source of this amino acid.

However, if you wish to include more in your diet then supplementation can be considered or an increase in foods containing phenylalanine which include:

Pasta

Oatmeal

Beef

Tuna and fish in general

Pork chops

Bacon

Soya

Tofu

Pinto beans

Milk

Nuts

You can see that a varied died should provide enough phenylalanine but clearly poor dietary habits –picking at food, older age which inhibits absorption, malabsorption due to inflammatory bowel disease, among others, can prevent optimal amounts of vital nutrients reaching their target.

The recommended daily intake is:

25mg/kg/daily.

Octacosanol

Octacosanol is a chemical found in many plants including sugar cane. It is also found in wheat germ. It is very similar to vitamin E.

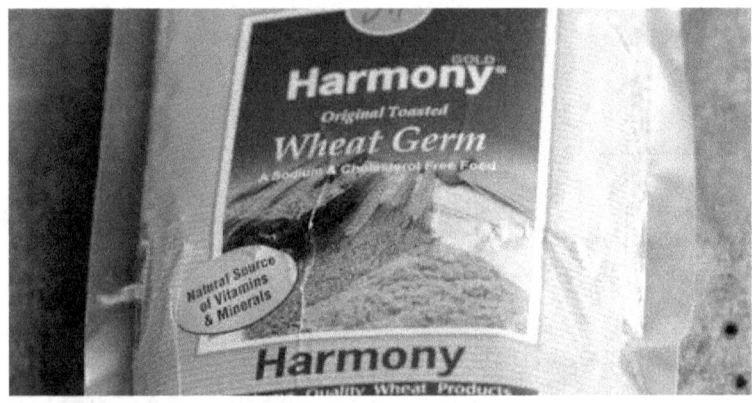

Octacosanol is known for improving exercise performance as well as stamina and strength.

It has been used to improve Parkinson's disease and amyotrophic lateral sclerosis (Lou Gehrig's disease) and arteriosclerosis which is the hardening of the arteries as opposed to atherosclerosis which is where plaque blocks the arteries.

Octacosanol appears to enhance the way that our body uses oxygen. In an experimental study,[15] 10 patients with mild to moderate symptoms randomly received Octacosanol in a wheat germ oil base at 5mg 3 times daily with meals or a placebo for 6 weeks only.

A standard self-appraisal form was used. 3/10 significantly improved and none worsened on the octacosanol. The experimental group showed a small but significant improvement in activities of daily living and mood ratings when compared to the placebo group

---

[15] Snider SR. Octacosanol in parkinsonism. Ann. Neurology 16:723, 1984

In conclusion, studies spanning decades have shown that bespoke nutrition can slow down the progression of Parkinson's disease and, in many cases, remove the symptoms. Knowing this gives the patient greater control over their life and condition. L- dopa has many distressing side effects and if, by judicious planning of meals and supplementation, the dosage of L-dopa can be reduced then this is all to the good.

This book will, hopefully, set those with Parkinson's disease on a new journey of hope.

Therapeutic cake for those with Parkinson's disease

This cake is easy to make but specifically, it adds nutrients which are known to help those with Parkinson's disease. Additionally, it can help reverse or slow down the symptoms of osteoporosis. As all the ingredients are important in their own right, please try not to leave any out. A slice of cake is a meal in itself but benefits increase if the cake is spread with a little malt or eaten with a banana.

The supplements need to be ground down in a coffee grinder if you are unable to find them in powder form. They then need to be soaked in a little milk for 30 minutes before adding to the mixture.

You must use fava flour instead of wheat flour as fava flour increases Levodopa and alleviates the symptoms better than prescription medicine.

Ingredients

2 eggs beaten

Fava flour to bind so quantity will vary

Honey to taste

50g of powdered milk

4 ounces of ground almonds

4 brazil nuts chopped finely

½ lb dried fruit of choice

20 000 IU's of vitamin D in powder form soaked in a little milk

100mg of powdered zinc soaked in a little milk

1 or 2 apples finely grated

Spice if desired, of choice

½ teaspoon of bicarbonate of soda

Method

Melt the butter and allow to cool slightly

Tip all the ingredients into a large bowl with the melted butter, apart from the fava flour. Mix well.

Add fava flour until the cake mixture is not too wet and sloppy and is bound well.

Line a cake tin with greaseproof and spoon the mixture in, smoothing down the top. Allow to settle for 15 minutes. Place in a heated oven at 170C. Watch the top of the cake and if it looks as though it is going to burn then lay over some aluminium.

Depending on how wet the cake was, check the cake after 40 minutes by inserting a knife into the mixture. If there is some uncooked mixture clinging to the knife, then return the cake to the oven for a further 20-30minutes. Repeat this as often as necessary.

When cooked allow to cool   before removing from the tin but take the greaseproof off before   the cake has entirely cooled otherwise it will stick to the cake

The cake can be cut into slices and frozen. It is nutritionally dense.

Broad Bean Pate

450g broad beans – frozen or fresh

1 clove garlic

7 sprigs of fresh mint

Some parsley to taste

90ml of olive oil

Method

Cook the beans in as little water as possible but reserve the water left over.

Blitz all the ingredients together until smooth using some of the reserve water to help blend.

Leave for 30 minutes to allow flavours to blend.

Table showing the nutritional benefits of food items relevant to Parkinson's Disease

Food item	Nutritional substance	benefits
Nuts, nut milk and nut butters	Myo-inositol	properties include a remarkable ability to enhance the clearance of disease proteins, which has obvious therapeutic possibilities in all protein aggregation diseases, including Alzheimer's, Parkinson's Disease, Lewy Body Dementia and Motor Neuron Disease.
Peas and all types of beans including kidney,	Myo-inositol	See above

butter and pinto beans Fava beans (broad beans)	tyrosine	Increases Levodopa as well as providing myo-inositol
Whole-wheat cereals like all bran, Weetabix (bear in mind that due to the added niacin in Weetabix, this sometimes causes indigestion and should be stopped if it does as inositol can be obtained from other sources	Myo-inositol	See above
Liver but particularly chicken liver and pates made from liver	Myo-inositol	As above
Citrus fruits and melon	Myo-inositol	As above
Fresh fruit and lightly cooked vegetables as prolonged	Vitamin C	Vitamin C deficiency is associated with

| cooking would destroy the vitamin C | | Parkinsonism symptoms |

Insulin resistance is a complex condition in which the body doesn't respond to insulin.

There appears to be a link with insulin resistance and Parkinson's disease as well as other neurodegenerative disorders.

Insulin is necessary to help use up glucose in the bloodstream by allowing the cells in muscles, liver and fat to take it up and use it.

Insulin resistance occurs as a result of genetic and lifestyle factors.

HOW DOES INSULIN WORK?

All food which is eaten is broken down into glucose (sugar). This is the main source of energy for the body.

When the glucose enters your bloodstream, it signals your pancreas to   release insulin.

Insulin helps the glucose enter muscle, fat and liver cells so it can be used for energy immediately or stored in fat cells for later use.

When glucose has entered the cells, there is less in the bloodstream and this is a signal for the pancreas to stop producing insulin.

Sometimes, the cells in muscle, fat and liver do not respond properly to insulin and they are not very efficient in taking up insulin. This is called insulin resistance.

As the cells aren't taking up the glucose, the body senses the extra glucose in the bloodstream and releases even more insulin.

This excessive release of insulin is known as hyperinsulinemia.

If the pancreas can respond to the need for extra insulin, everything is OK but if not then prediabetes, type2 diabetes and high blood sugar levels occur.

Insulin resistance is associated with many conditions such as obesity, non-alcoholic fatty liver disease, metabolic syndrome, cardiovascular disease, polycystic ovary syndrome and infertility problems, as well as Parkinson's disease. It is associated with high blood pressure and hardening of the arteries.

The 'healthy' oils like sunflower and rapeseed oil also increase the potential for insulin resistance and should be avoided in favour of the non-inflammatory animal fats.

Insulin resistance is associated with increased thirst

Increased peeing

Increased hunger

Headaches and blurred vision

Skin infections

However, the above symptoms do not need to be present all at the same time for insulin resistance to be present.

The popular Keto diet appears to be the way forward in treating insulin resistance.

The keto diet relies on most of the calories in food being obtained mainly from fat and not carbohydrates with proper protein intake clearly being an important factor. It is not easy to give definitive protein needs for any age group as this is also dependent on environmental factors including how active the person is. While guides are available on the internet, they are only guides and if someone fancies a four egg omelette with 3 rashes of bacon at any time, I cannot see why this would be a problem.

The keto diet allows you to eat generously of sources of animal protein, animal fat and unlimited green leafy veg. Nuts are also useful on the keto diet as they do not contain a great deal of carbohydrate and there is no preparation apart from opening the bag. Further, they contain the much coveted inositol.

However, caution with any nut needs to be exercised. Tiny pieces tend to get caught in the throat even in people without the swallowing problem found in those with neurodegenerative disorders.

Soaking nuts before adding to muesli, using nut flours in cakes, grinding them up and adding them to melted chocolate for a decadent bite are all useful tips. It is quite possible to add a teaspoon of inositol to the mix and it won't impair the flavour.

Recipes for Parkinson's Disease

These foods **do not act like pharmaceutical MAO-B inhibitors**, but they contain compounds (kaempferol, apigenin, quercetin, epicatechin, luteolin, curcumin, piperine, etc.) that have been studied for **neuroprotective, antioxidant, anti-inflammatory, and mitochondrial-supportive effects**, which may complement Parkinson's care.

20 Recipes Featuring Natural MAO-B–Relevant Compounds

1. Turmeric–Ginger Golden Milk

Key compounds: Curcumin, fragrant ginger (galangal), piperine
Ingredients

- 1 cup milk or plant milk
- ½ tsp turmeric
- ¼ tsp ground galangal or fresh ginger
- Pinch black pepper
- ½ tsp honey

Method Warm everything gently for 5 minutes; do not boil.

Why beneficial
Curcumin is poorly absorbed unless paired with piperine; this combination increases bioavailability and

supports anti-inflammatory pathways relevant to neuroprotection.

2. Coffee–Cinnamon Morning Smoothie

Key compounds: Coffee polyphenols, quercetin (from berries)
Ingredients

- 1 shot cooled espresso
- ½ cup blueberries
- ½ banana
- ½ cup milk or yoghurt
- Pinch cinnamon

Method Blend until smooth.

Why beneficial
Coffee contains compounds associated with reduced Parkinson's risk; berries add quercetin and anthocyanins that support neuronal resilience.

3. Ginger–Galangal Stir-Fry Vegetables

Key compounds: Kaempferol (greens), galangal
Ingredients

- 2 cups mixed greens (kale, spinach)
- 1 tbsp grated galangal
- 1 tbsp grated ginger
- 1 tbsp olive oil

- Splash tamari

Method Sauté ginger/galangal, add greens, cook 3–4 minutes.

Why beneficial
Leafy greens are rich in kaempferol, a flavonoid studied for MAO-B modulation and antioxidant effects.

4. Curried Lentil Soup with Turmeric & Ginger

Key compounds: Curcumin, apigenin (celery), luteolin (carrots)
Ingredients

- 1 cup red lentils
- 1 carrot, diced
- 1 celery stalk
- 1 tsp turmeric
- 1 tsp grated ginger
- 1 tsp curry powder

Method Simmer all ingredients 20 minutes.

Why beneficial
Combines curcumin with apigenin-rich celery and luteolin-rich carrots for broad anti-inflammatory support.

5. Dark Chocolate & Berry Bowl

Key compounds: Epicatechin (dark chocolate), quercetin (berries)
Ingredients

- 20–30 g dark chocolate (70%+)
- ½ cup mixed berries
- 1 tbsp chopped nuts

Method Melt chocolate lightly, drizzle over berries.

Why beneficial
Epicatechin supports mitochondrial function; quercetin adds antioxidant and anti-aggregation effects.

6. Nutmeg-Spiced Overnight Oats

Key compounds: Nutmeg, quercetin (apples)
Ingredients

- ½ cup oats
- ½ cup milk
- ½ grated apple
- Pinch nutmeg
- Pinch cinnamon

Method Combine and refrigerate overnight.

Why beneficial
Nutmeg contains compounds with mild MAO-B–modulating potential; oats and apples add steady glucose support.

7. Liquorice Root Tea

Key compounds: Liquorice flavonoids
Ingredients

- 1 tsp dried liquorice root
- 1 cup hot water

Method Steep 10 minutes.

Why beneficial
Liquorice contains glabridin, studied for neuroprotective antioxidant effects.

(Note: avoid in hypertension.)

8. Quercetin-Rich Apple–Onion Sauté

Key compounds: Quercetin (onions, apples)
Ingredients

- 1 sliced onion
- 1 sliced apple
- 1 tbsp olive oil

Method Sauté onions until soft, add apples, cook 5 minutes.

Why beneficial
Onions are one of the richest quercetin sources; gentle cooking preserves flavonoids.

9. Luteolin-Boosted Herb Omelette

Key compounds: Luteolin (parsley), apigenin (chamomile tea on the side)
Ingredients

- 2 eggs
- Handful chopped parsley
- Salt & pepper

Method Whisk eggs, add parsley, cook gently.

Why beneficial
Parsley is a potent luteolin source; luteolin is studied for microglial calming and anti-inflammatory effects.

10. Ginger–Turmeric Carrot Soup

Key compounds: Curcumin, luteolin (carrots), gingerols
Ingredients

- 4 carrots
- 1 tsp turmeric
- 1 tsp ginger
- 2 cups stock

Method Simmer 20 minutes, blend.

Why beneficial
Carrots add luteolin; turmeric and ginger support anti-inflammatory pathways.

11. Galangal & Coconut Fish Curry

Key compounds: Kaempferol (greens), galangal, curcumin
Ingredients

- 1 tbsp grated galangal
- 1 tsp turmeric
- 1 can coconut milk
- White fish fillets
- Handful spinach

Method Simmer spices in coconut milk, add fish, finish with spinach.

Why beneficial
Galangal contains kaempferol derivatives; turmeric adds curcumin for neuroinflammation support.

12. Black Pepper–Turmeric Roasted Cauliflower

Key compounds: Curcumin + piperine synergy
Ingredients

- 1 cauliflower
- 1 tsp turmeric
- ½ tsp black pepper
- 1 tbsp olive oil

Method Roast 25 minutes at 200°C.

Why beneficial
Piperine enhances curcumin absorption dramatically; cauliflower adds sulforaphane-related compounds.

13. Apigenin-Rich Chamomile Poached Pears

Key compounds: Apigenin (chamomile)
Ingredients

- 2 pears
- 1 cup strong chamomile tea
- 1 tbsp honey

Method Simmer pears in chamomile tea until soft.

Why beneficial
Apigenin is a gentle flavonoid with anxiolytic and neuroprotective properties.

14. Dark Chocolate–Nutmeg Truffles

Key compounds: Epicatechin, nutmeg
Ingredients

- 100 g dark chocolate
- 2 tbsp cream
- Pinch nutmeg

Method Melt chocolate, stir in cream and nutmeg, chill and roll.

Why beneficial
Epicatechin supports neuronal energy metabolism; nutmeg adds additional flavonoids.

15. Ginger–Lemon Herbal Shot

Key compounds: Gingerols, galangal (optional)
Ingredients

- 1 tbsp grated ginger
- ½ tsp grated galangal
- Juice of ½ lemon
- Warm water

Method Mix and drink fresh.

Why beneficial
Ginger and galangal support antioxidant pathways and may reduce neuroinflammation.

16. Curcumin–Piperine Hummus

Key compounds: Curcumin, piperine
Ingredients

- 1 can chickpeas
- 1 tsp turmeric
- ¼ tsp black pepper
- 1 tbsp tahini
- Lemon juice

Method Blend all ingredients.

Why beneficial
A savoury way to combine curcumin with its absorption enhancer.

17. Quercetin-Boosted Red Onion & Tomato Salad

Key compounds: Quercetin (red onion), kaempferol (greens)
Ingredients

- ½ red onion
- 2 tomatoes
- Handful rocket or spinach
- Olive oil & lemon

Method Slice and dress.

Why beneficial
Raw red onion is one of the richest quercetin sources.

18. Liquorice-Spiced Carrot & Ginger Bake

Key compounds: Liquorice, luteolin (carrots), ginger
Ingredients

- 4 carrots
- ½ tsp liquorice powder
- 1 tsp grated ginger
- Olive oil

Method Roast 25 minutes.

Why beneficial
Liquorice adds glabridin; carrots add luteolin for microglial calming.

19. Coffee-Rubbed Chicken

Key compounds: Coffee polyphenols, piperine
Ingredients

- 1 tbsp ground coffee
- ½ tsp black pepper
- 1 tsp paprika
- Chicken breasts

Method Rub chicken with spices, bake 20 minutes.

Why beneficial
Coffee polyphenols have antioxidant and neuroprotective associations; pepper adds piperine.

20. Galangal–Turmeric Vegetable Broth

Key compounds: Kaempferol (greens), curcumin, galangal
Ingredients

- 1 tsp turmeric
- 1 tbsp sliced galangal
- 1 carrot

- 1 celery stalk
- Handful greens
- 1 litre water

Method Simmer 30 minutes.

Why beneficial
A gentle, daily-use broth combining multiple flavonoids with anti-inflammatory potential.

10 Recipes High in Thiamine (B1) & Vitamin B6

1. Salmon, Spinach & Sunflower Seed Bowl

Ingredients

- 1 salmon fillet
- 2 cups spinach
- 2 tbsp sunflower seeds
- ½ cup cooked brown rice
- Lemon, olive oil

Method
Bake salmon 12–15 minutes. Wilt spinach in a pan. Assemble bowl with rice, spinach, salmon, and seeds.

Why beneficial
Salmon is rich in B6; sunflower seeds and brown rice add thiamine.

2. Chickpea & Potato Curry

Ingredients

- 1 can chickpeas
- 2 potatoes, diced
- 1 onion
- 1 tsp turmeric
- 1 tsp curry powder
- 1 cup coconut milk

Method
Sauté onion, add spices, potatoes, chickpeas, and coconut milk. Simmer 20 minutes.

Why beneficial
Chickpeas and potatoes provide both B1 and B6; onions add extra B6.

3. Chicken & Lentil Stew

Ingredients

- 1 chicken breast, diced
- 1 cup red lentils
- 1 carrot
- 1 celery stalk

- 1 tsp paprika

Method
Brown chicken, add vegetables and lentils, cover with water, simmer 25 minutes.

Why beneficial
Chicken is high in B6; lentils contribute thiamine and additional B6.

4. Wholegrain Toast with Avocado, Egg & Nutritional Yeast

Ingredients

- 1–2 slices wholegrain bread
- 1 boiled or poached egg
- ½ avocado
- 1 tbsp nutritional yeast

Method
Toast bread, mash avocado, top with egg and nutritional yeast.

Why beneficial
Whole grains and nutritional yeast are excellent thiamine sources; eggs add B6.

5. Banana–Oat Breakfast Muffins

Ingredients

- 2 ripe bananas
- 1 cup oats
- 1 egg
- 1 tbsp honey
- ½ tsp cinnamon

Method
Mash bananas, mix all ingredients, bake 15 minutes at 180°C.

Why beneficial
Bananas provide B6; oats contribute thiamine.

6. Black Bean & Sweet Potato Burrito Bowl

Ingredients

- 1 cup cooked black beans
- 1 roasted sweet potato
- ½ cup brown rice
- Salsa or lime

Method
Assemble bowl with rice, beans, sweet potato, and toppings.

Why beneficial
Black beans are rich in thiamine; sweet potatoes add B6.

7. Tuna, Egg & Spinach Salad

Ingredients

- 1 can tuna
- 2 boiled eggs
- 2 cups spinach
- Olive oil & lemon

Method
Combine all ingredients and dress lightly.

Why beneficial
Tuna and eggs provide B6; spinach adds thiamine and additional B vitamins.

8. Sunflower Seed & Lentil Patties

Ingredients

- 1 cup cooked lentils
- ¼ cup sunflower seeds
- 1 grated carrot
- 1 egg
- 1 tbsp flour

Method
Mix ingredients, form patties, pan-fry 3 minutes per side.

Why beneficial
Lentils and sunflower seeds are strong thiamine sources; carrot and egg add B6.

9. Brown Rice Stir-Fry with Tofu & Vegetables

Ingredients

- 1 cup cooked brown rice
- ½ block tofu
- 1 cup mixed vegetables (broccoli, peppers)
- Tamari or soy sauce

Method
Stir-fry tofu, add vegetables, then rice and tamari.

Why beneficial
Brown rice provides thiamine; tofu and vegetables contribute B6.

10. Sardine & Tomato Wholegrain Pasta

Ingredients

- 1 tin sardines
- 1 cup wholegrain pasta
- 1 cup cherry tomatoes
- Garlic, olive oil

Method
Cook pasta, sauté tomatoes and garlic, add sardines, toss together.

Why beneficial
Sardines are rich in B6; wholegrain pasta adds thiamine.

10 Recipes to Increase Magnesium

1. Spinach, Avocado & Pumpkin Seed Salad

Ingredients

- 2 cups fresh spinach
- ½ avocado, sliced
- 2 tbsp pumpkin seeds
- 1 tbsp olive oil
- Lemon juice

Method
Assemble ingredients and dress lightly.

Why beneficial
Spinach and pumpkin seeds are two of the richest natural magnesium sources; avocado adds more plus healthy fats.

2. Black Bean & Brown Rice Bowl

Ingredients

- 1 cup cooked black beans
- ½ cup cooked brown rice
- 1 tomato, chopped
- Lime juice
- Fresh coriander

Method
Warm beans, combine with rice and toppings.

Why beneficial
Black beans and brown rice both provide magnesium and steady energy.

3. Almond–Banana Overnight Oats

Ingredients

- ½ cup oats
- 1 cup milk or plant milk
- 1 banana, sliced
- 2 tbsp almonds (whole or chopped)

Method
Mix oats and milk, refrigerate overnight, top with banana and almonds.

Why beneficial
Oats and almonds are magnesium-dense; bananas add additional B vitamins and potassium.

4. Dark Chocolate & Nut Trail Mix

Ingredients

- ¼ cup almonds
- ¼ cup cashews
- ¼ cup pumpkin seeds

- 20 g dark chocolate (70%+)

Method
Combine all ingredients.

Why beneficial
Pumpkin seeds and almonds are magnesium powerhouses; dark chocolate adds extra magnesium and polyphenols.

5. Tofu & Vegetable Stir-Fry

Ingredients

- ½ block firm tofu, cubed
- 1 cup broccoli florets
- 1 cup spinach
- 1 tbsp tamari
- 1 tsp sesame oil

Method
Stir-fry tofu until golden, add vegetables, finish with tamari.

Why beneficial
Tofu and leafy greens contribute significant magnesium; broccoli adds supportive minerals.

6. Creamy Chickpea & Spinach Soup

Ingredients

- 1 can chickpeas
- 2 cups spinach
- 1 onion
- 2 cups vegetable stock
- 1 tsp cumin

Method
Sauté onion, add chickpeas, stock, and spinach; simmer 10 minutes and blend.

Why beneficial
Chickpeas and spinach both deliver magnesium and fibre.

7. Avocado, Black Bean & Corn Wrap

Ingredients

- 1 wholegrain wrap
- ½ avocado
- ½ cup black beans
- ¼ cup sweetcorn
- Lime & pepper

Method
Layer ingredients in the wrap and fold.

Why beneficial
Black beans and avocado provide magnesium; wholegrain wraps add more.

8. Salmon with Almond–Herb Crust

Ingredients

- 1 salmon fillet
- 2 tbsp crushed almonds
- 1 tsp lemon zest
- Pinch herbs

Method
Press almond mixture onto salmon and bake 12–15 minutes.

Why beneficial
Almonds are magnesium-rich; salmon adds omega-3s that support neurological health.

9. Quinoa, Spinach & Chickpea Pilaf

Ingredients

- 1 cup cooked quinoa
- 1 cup chickpeas
- 2 cups spinach
- 1 tbsp olive oil
- Garlic (optional)

Method
Sauté garlic, add spinach, stir in quinoa and chickpeas.

Why beneficial
Quinoa and chickpeas both contain magnesium; spinach boosts the total significantly.

10. Baked Sweet Potato with Tahini & Pumpkin Seeds

Ingredients

- 1 sweet potato
- 1 tbsp tahini
- 1 tbsp pumpkin seeds

Method
Bake sweet potato until soft, top with tahini and seeds.

Why beneficial
Pumpkin seeds and tahini (sesame paste) are exceptionally high in magnesium.

Glabridin: What It Is and Why It Matters

What is glabridin?

Glabridin is a **natural flavonoid** found in the root of *Glycyrrhiza glabra* — the plant commonly known as **liquorice**.
It belongs to a group of plant compounds called **isoflavans**, which act as antioxidants and cell-protective agents. Glabridin is one of the main active components in liquorice root extract and is responsible for many of its biological effects.

Why glabridin is considered beneficial

1. Powerful antioxidant support

Glabridin helps neutralise **oxidative stress**, one of the major drivers of:

- cellular ageing
- inflammation
- mitochondrial strain
- neuronal vulnerability

This antioxidant activity is one of the reasons it appears in discussions about neuroprotection.

2. Anti-inflammatory effects

Glabridin can calm inflammatory signalling pathways. This matters because chronic inflammation contributes to:

- neurodegenerative processes
- metabolic imbalance
- vascular stress

By reducing inflammatory load, glabridin may help create a more stable internal environment.

3. Potential neuroprotective actions

Early research suggests glabridin may help protect nerve cells by:

- reducing oxidative injury
- supporting mitochondrial energy production
- moderating overactive microglia (the brain's immune cells)

These mechanisms are relevant to long-term brain health and resilience.

4. Gentle hormone-modulating activity

Glabridin has mild **phytoestrogen-like** effects.
This doesn't act like medication, but it may support:

- cognitive function
- vascular health
- metabolic stability

Its activity is subtle and food-level, not pharmaceutical.

5. Cardiovascular support

Liquorice flavonoids, including glabridin, have been studied for:

- supporting healthy cholesterol balance
- protecting blood vessels from oxidative stress
- improving endothelial function

These effects contribute to overall metabolic and vascular wellbeing.

6. Additional benefits

Outside neurology, glabridin is also used for:

- calming skin inflammation
- reducing pigmentation
- supporting glucose metabolism

These show its broad biological activity.

Safety note

Liquorice root naturally contains **glycyrrhizin**, which can raise blood pressure in some people.
Glabridin itself is not the issue, but whole liquorice products vary widely.

For culinary use:

- **small amounts are generally safe**
- people with **hypertension** should avoid concentrated liquorice extracts unless advised otherwise

Food-Based Ways to Include Glabridin (Liquorice Flavonoids) Safely

Glabridin comes from **liquorice root**, not the black confectionery sweets.
Culinary use is mild, flavour-focused, and avoids the high glycyrrhizin levels found in strong extracts.

Below are **safe, kitchen-level ways** to incorporate liquorice root into recipes without drifting into therapeutic dosing.

1. Liquorice Root Herbal Tea

How to use:
Simmer 1 tsp dried liquorice root in hot water for 10 minutes.

Why this works:
A gentle infusion releases glabridin and other flavonoids without excessive glycyrrhizin.

2. Liquorice-Spiced Carrot Soup

How to use:
Add ¼–½ tsp liquorice root powder while sautéing onions and carrots.

Why this works:
Carrots bring luteolin; liquorice adds glabridin for a warm, subtly sweet depth.

3. Liquorice & Ginger Broth

How to use:
Add a small piece of dried liquorice root to a pot of vegetable or chicken broth; remove before serving.

Why this works:
Infuses flavour and flavonoids without overpowering the dish.

4. Liquorice-Infused Porridge

How to use:
Simmer oats with a tiny pinch of liquorice powder and cinnamon.

Why this works:
Oats provide steady glucose support; liquorice adds antioxidant compounds.

5. Spiced Roasted Nuts with Liquorice

How to use:
Toss almonds or cashews with olive oil, a pinch of liquorice powder, and paprika; roast lightly.

Why this works:
Nuts add magnesium and healthy fats; liquorice contributes glabridin.

6. Liquorice-Orange Herbal Syrup (Culinary, Not Medicinal)

How to use:
Simmer orange peel, a small liquorice root piece, and honey in water; use 1–2 tsp to flavour yoghurt or porridge.

Why this works:
Creates a gentle aromatic infusion with minimal glycyrrhizin.

7. Liquorice-Spiced Lentils

How to use:
Add a tiny pinch of liquorice powder to red lentils with turmeric and cumin.

Why this works:
Lentils provide B vitamins and minerals; liquorice adds flavonoids and warmth.

8. Liquorice & Apple Compote

How to use:
Simmer chopped apples with a small piece of liquorice root and a splash of water.

Why this works:
Apples bring quercetin; liquorice adds glabridin and a subtle sweetness.

9. Liquorice-Cocoa Hot Drink

How to use:
Add a pinch of liquorice powder to hot cocoa made with dark chocolate.

Why this works:
Dark chocolate provides epicatechin; liquorice adds complementary antioxidant activity.

10. Liquorice-Spiced Vegetable Bake

How to use:
Sprinkle a tiny amount of liquorice powder over carrots, parsnips, or sweet potatoes before roasting.

Why this works:
Root vegetables pair naturally with liquorice's warm, aromatic notes.

Appendix

Phytochemicals for Parkinson's

Curcumin

Food sources: Turmeric, curry blends
Why relevant: Antioxidant; anti-inflammatory; supports mitochondrial stability

Piperine
Food sources: Black pepper
Why relevant: Enhances curcumin absorption; antioxidant activity

Quercetin
Food sources: Red onions, apples, berries, kale
Why relevant: Potent antioxidant; supports mitochondrial enzymes

Kaempferol
Food sources: Spinach, kale, broccoli, green tea
Why relevant: Antioxidant; anti-inflammatory; mild MAO-B interest

Luteolin
Food sources: Parsley, celery, carrots, chamomile
Why relevant: Strong microglial-calming effects; anti-inflammatory

Apigenin
Food sources: Chamomile, parsley, celery, oregano
Why relevant: Gentle neuro-calming; antioxidant

Epicatechin
Food sources: Dark chocolate, green tea, black tea
Why relevant: Supports mitochondria; improves blood flow

Glabridin
Food sources: Liquorice root (culinary amounts)
Why relevant: Antioxidant; anti-inflammatory; mitochondrial support

Coffee Polyphenols
Food sources: Coffee, green tea, black tea
Why relevant: Linked with lower PD risk; mitochondrial support

Gingerols & Galangin
Food sources: Ginger, galangal
Why relevant: Anti-inflammatory; antioxidant; digestive support

Resveratrol
Food sources: Red grapes, blueberries, peanuts
Why relevant: Mitochondrial support; antioxidant

Sulforaphane Precursors
Food sources: Broccoli sprouts, broccoli, kale
Why relevant: Activates Nrf2 (master antioxidant switch)

What "Activates Nrf2 (master antioxidant switch)" Means

1. Nrf2 is your body's internal 'switch' for antioxidant defence

Nrf2 (pronounced *nerf-two*) is a **protein inside your cells**.
Its job is to act like a **master switch** that turns on hundreds of your body's own antioxidant and detoxification genes.

Think of it as the **control panel** for your natural defence system.

When Nrf2 is activated, your cells start producing:

- glutathione
- superoxide dismutase
- catalase
- detox enzymes
- anti-inflammatory proteins

These are far more powerful than anything you can get from food alone.

2. Why this matters for Parkinson's

Parkinson's involves:

- oxidative stress
- mitochondrial strain

- inflammation in the brain
- vulnerability of dopamine-producing neurons

Nrf2 activation helps counter these pressures by:

- reducing oxidative damage
- supporting mitochondrial resilience
- calming inflammatory signalling
- improving cellular clean-up processes

It doesn't treat Parkinson's, but it supports the **cellular environment** that neurons prefer.

3. How Nrf2 works

Under normal conditions, Nrf2 is kept "switched off" in the cell.

When certain plant compounds appear — like sulforaphane, curcumin, or resveratrol — they **release** Nrf2 so it can move into the nucleus and switch on protective genes.

It's like:

- the cell senses stress
- Nrf2 is released
- Nrf2 turns on the antioxidant machinery
- the cell becomes more resilient

4. Foods that activate Nrf2

These are the most studied:

- **Broccoli sprouts** (strongest natural source)
- Broccoli, kale, cabbage
- Turmeric (curcumin)
- Green tea
- Dark berries
- Ginger
- Garlic
- Resveratrol foods (grapes, blueberries, peanuts)

This is why broccoli sprouts often appear in neuroprotection discussions.

5. Why people call it the "master antioxidant switch"

Because Nrf2 doesn't just increase one antioxidant — it increases **dozens** at once.
It's like upgrading the whole system rather than adding one supplement.

Top Food Sources That Activate Nrf2 (Master Antioxidant Switch)

Broccoli sprouts
Highest natural source of sulforaphane, the strongest known dietary Nrf2 activator.

Broccoli
Reliable sulforaphane precursor; gentler than sprouts but still effective.

Kale
Rich in glucoraphanin (sulforaphane precursor) and other Nrf2-supportive compounds.

Cabbage and Brussels sprouts
Contain the same glucosinolate family that activates Nrf2.

Garlic
Contains organosulfur compounds that stimulate Nrf2 pathways.

Turmeric (curcumin)
Supports Nrf2 activation and reduces oxidative stress.

Green tea
EGCG helps activate Nrf2 and supports mitochondrial function.

Dark berries (blueberries, blackberries)
Anthocyanins support Nrf2 and reduce inflammation.

Ginger
Gingerols help activate Nrf2 and support detoxification pathways.

Resveratrol foods (grapes, blueberries, peanuts)
Support Nrf2 and mitochondrial biogenesis.

Mustard powder
A tiny pinch added to cooked broccoli restores STEP 1
— Nrf2 is "asleep"

Inside every cell, Nrf2 is kept switched off and held in place by a protein called Keap1.

STEP 2 — A trigger appears

Certain plant compounds (sulforaphane, curcumin, green tea polyphenols, garlic compounds, resveratrol)

cause mild, healthy stress signals inside the cell.

STEP 3 — Nrf2 is released

These signals loosen Nrf2 from Keap1, allowing it to move freely.

STEP 4 — Nrf2 enters the nucleus

Nrf2 travels into the cell's nucleus — the control centre where genes are switched on or off.

STEP 5 — Nrf2 switches on protective genes

Once inside the nucleus, Nrf2 activates hundreds of genes responsible for:

- antioxidant enzymes (glutathione, SOD, catalase)

- detoxification enzymes

- anti-inflammatory proteins

- mitochondrial protection

- cellular clean-up and repair

STEP 6 — The cell becomes more resilient

With these genes activated, the cell is better able to:

- neutralise oxidative stress

- reduce inflammation

- protect mitochondria

- clear damaged proteins

- maintain long-term function

This is why Nrf2 is called the "master antioxidant switch."sulforaphane formation.

Why Protein Timing Matters for Levodopa

People often notice that their Parkinson's medication works brilliantly some days and less well on others. One of the most common everyday reasons is **protein timing**.

Here's the simple explanation:

1. Levodopa and protein use the same "transport system"

Inside the gut and across the blood–brain barrier, levodopa and certain amino acids from protein share the **same transport channels**.
If both arrive at the same time, they compete.

2. When protein "wins," less levodopa gets through

This doesn't harm you — it just means:

- the medication may take longer to work
- the effect may feel weaker
- "off" periods may appear sooner

It's not the protein itself that's the problem — it's the **timing**.

3. Spacing protein and levodopa helps the medication get where it needs to go

Many people find that having their main protein-rich meals **later in the day** or **away from medication times** helps their levodopa feel more consistent.

This is not a rule or a restriction — just a **practical pattern** that some people find useful.

4. Everyone is different

Some people are very sensitive to protein timing.
Others notice no difference at all.
It's simply one of the everyday factors that can influence how levodopa feels.

5. This is not about eating less protein

Protein is essential for:

- muscle strength
- immune function
- energy
- healing

The goal is not to reduce protein — just to understand how timing can affect medication absorption.

Glossary (Alphabetical Order)

Amino acids
The building blocks of protein. Some of them use the same transport pathways as levodopa.

Antioxidant
A substance that helps protect cells from everyday metabolic stress and damage.

Blood–brain barrier
A protective layer that controls what can enter the brain from the bloodstream.

Constipation
A common symptom in Parkinson's that can affect comfort and how well medication is absorbed.

Dopamine
A chemical messenger involved in movement, motivation, and mood. In Parkinson's, the brain gradually makes less of it.

Flavonoids
Plant compounds found in fruits, vegetables, herbs, and teas. Many have antioxidant and anti-inflammatory effects.

Glabridin
A flavonoid from liquorice root with antioxidant and anti-inflammatory properties.

Gut–brain axis
The communication network between the digestive system and the brain.

Inflammation
The body's response to stress or injury. Chronic inflammation can affect brain health.

Levodopa
A medication that the body converts into dopamine. It helps improve movement and reduce stiffness.

MAO-B
An enzyme that breaks down dopamine. Some plant compounds have mild, natural interactions with this pathway.

Microglia
The brain's immune cells. When over-activated, they can contribute to inflammation.

Mitochondria
The energy-producing parts of cells. They help keep neurons functioning.

Nrf2
A protein inside cells that switches on the body's own antioxidant and detoxification systems.

Oxidative stress
A type of cellular "wear and tear" caused by unstable molecules called free radicals.

Polyphenols
A large family of plant compounds (including flavonoids) that support cellular resilience.

Sulforaphane
A compound formed from cruciferous vegetables (especially broccoli sprouts) that activates Nrf2.

Vitamins and Their Key Activators / Co-Factors

B1 (Thiamine)

Helps with: energy production, nerve function
Key activators / co-factors:

- Magnesium
- Sulphur-containing foods (garlic, onions)
- Manganese
- Vitamin C (supports regeneration)

B2 (Riboflavin)

Helps with: mitochondrial energy, antioxidant recycling
Key activators / co-factors:

- Magnesium
- Selenium
- Iron (for proper utilisation)
- B3 (they work in the same pathways)

B3 (Niacin / NAD pathways)

Helps with: mitochondrial energy, DNA repair
Key activators / co-factors:

- Tryptophan (amino acid precursor)
- B2 and B6 (needed for conversion)
- Magnesium

- Iron

B5 (Pantothenic Acid)

Helps with: adrenal support, energy metabolism
Key activators / co-factors:

- Magnesium
- Vitamin C
- B2 and B3 (shared pathways)

B6 (Pyridoxine / P5P)

Helps with: neurotransmitter formation, amino acid metabolism
Key activators / co-factors:

- Magnesium (essential for activation to P5P)
- Zinc
- B2 (required for conversion to active form)
- Protein (provides amino acids B6 works on)

B7 (Biotin)

Helps with: blood sugar regulation, fatty acid metabolism
Key activators / co-factors:

- Magnesium
- B5
- Sulphur-rich foods (biotin contains sulphur)

B9 (Folate)

Helps with: methylation, DNA repair, red blood cell formation
Key activators / co-factors:

- B12 (they work as a pair)
- Vitamin C (helps convert folate to active forms)
- Magnesium
- Zinc (supports folate enzymes)

B12 (Cobalamin)

Helps with: nerve health, red blood cells, methylation
Key activators / co-factors:

- Folate (B9)
- B6
- Magnesium
- Choline / betaine (methylation support)

B-Vitamins: What Inhibits or Destroys Them

B1 (Thiamine)

Inhibitors / destroyers:

- Alcohol
- High sugar intake
- Raw fish containing thiaminase

- Coffee and tea (tannins reduce absorption)
- Diuretics
- High-carbohydrate diets increase demand
- Chronic stress increases usage

B2 (Riboflavin)

Inhibitors / destroyers:

- **Sunlight** (riboflavin is light-sensitive)
- UV exposure
- Long cooking times
- Oral contraceptives
- Some antidepressants
- High alcohol intake

B3 (Niacin / NAD pathways)

Inhibitors / destroyers:

- Alcohol
- High sugar intake
- Oral contraceptives
- Stress (increases NAD turnover)
- Low protein intake (reduces tryptophan availability)

B5 (Pantothenic Acid)

Inhibitors / destroyers:

- Heat (easily destroyed by cooking)
- Alcohol
- Stress (increases adrenal demand)
- Oral contraceptives

B6 (Pyridoxine / P5P)

Inhibitors / destroyers:

- Alcohol
- Oral contraceptives
- Some anti-tuberculosis medications
- High-heat cooking
- Chronic inflammation increases demand
- Low magnesium (prevents activation to P5P)

B7 (Biotin)

Inhibitors / destroyers:

- Raw egg whites (contain avidin, which binds biotin)
- Alcohol
- Long-term antibiotics (affect gut bacteria that make biotin)

B9 (Folate)

Inhibitors / destroyers:

- Heat (folate is easily destroyed by cooking)
- Alcohol
- Smoking
- Oral contraceptives
- Some anti-seizure medications
- Low vitamin C (needed for activation)
- Gut issues affecting absorption

B12 (Cobalamin)

Inhibitors / destroyers:

- **PPI medications** (reduce stomach acid needed for absorption)
- **Metformin**
- Alcohol
- Smoking
- Low stomach acid (age-related or medication-related)
- Gut conditions affecting absorption

Foods Rich in Octacosanol

Wheat germ oil
The richest natural source of octacosanol. Even small amounts contain meaningful levels.

Wheat germ (raw or lightly heated)
Contains long-chain alcohols including octacosanol.

Sugarcane wax / unrefined sugarcane products
Naturally high in policosanols, including octacosanol.

Spinach
A reliable plant source; levels are lower than wheat germ oil but still significant.

Leafy greens (various)
Contain small amounts of long-chain alcohols that include octacosanol.

Whole grains
Trace amounts, especially in the outer layers of the grain.

How Octacosanol Supports Movement (Plain-English Explanation)

Octacosanol is a natural compound that seems to help the body use oxygen more efficiently during movement. Here's how it supports smoother, steadier physical function:

1. Helps muscles use oxygen more effectively
This can translate into better stamina and less fatigue during everyday activities.

2. Supports nerve signalling
Octacosanol appears to help nerve cells communicate more smoothly, which may contribute to steadier movement.

3. Reduces oxidative stress in muscles and nerves
By helping to neutralise everyday metabolic stress, octacosanol supports muscle recovery and cellular resilience.

4. May help coordination
Some early research suggests it can support smoother, more controlled movement patterns.

5. Naturally found in food
You don't need supplements — wheat germ oil, spinach, and sugarcane products provide it in a gentle, food-based form.

Other books by this author include:

- The EDS and Hypermobility Syndrome Diet
- Alleviating Symptoms of EDS
- Gastroparesis
- The EDS recipe book
- The Lipoedema Diet
- The Lymphoedema Diet: reverse and repair lymphatic damage
- The Anti Virus Diet
- The Asthma Diet
- The Reluctant Bowel
- The MND Diet
- Why we live longer with higher cholesterol levels
- A dietary connection for MACS, POTS and EDS
- Identity: a self-exploration workbook *
- Journey Through Pneumonia
- https://www.amazon.co.uk/dp/B07TBHMV6N

*This book can be used alone or in small group work and is an excellent resource for those who are 'people helpers.'

Among many others

They are available on Amazon

Lynne has written a semi-autobiographical trilogy.

For the full range of books by this author, visit the author website on

https://www.amazon.co.uk/-/e/B07BPQZ5CD

https://www.amazon.com/-/e/B07BPQZ5CD

A percentage of the profits from the sale of these books go to support charities like the Exodus Project below.

The Exodus Project

My first introduction to the far reaching impact of The Exodus Project occurred when I was travelling around Cawthorne in one of their buses, visiting gardens. A young lad was happily munching on a sandwich. He looked up briefly, pointed to the driver and said,' He's my second dad, he is,' then he returned to his sandwich without further comment

Such remarks are often very telling and so I arranged to meet Jackie Peel and Martin Sawdon, at the charity's premises in Barnsley. They set up the Exodus Project 20 years ago. They moved into their current premises – a redundant Methodist church - in 2010.

Both Jackie and Martin have been youth workers in their church. Martin worked in housing for the homeless in addition to working in learning disabilities services in institutional settings.

The work that the Exodus Project undertakes is of paramount importance to the communities it serves. These were former mining communities which became disadvantaged after pit-closures. Currently about 400 children attend mid-week activities from Monday to Thursday inclusive. These activities include dance, drama, craft, music, sports and games. In addition, there are weekend camps, cycle treks, outward bound activities, bowling and swimming. The children are taught valuable life skills including how to cook and bake. It is all about teaching children how to fulfil their potential and learn skills they will be able to pass onto the next generation.

The grounds, once overgrown, have been turned into a play- and camping - ground. A miniature railway is in the process of being installed.

Martin and Jackie have developed a unique model in that The Exodus Project goes beyond dispensing services. They are keen to build up relationships with the whole family and not just the child that attends the mid- week clubs. In addition, once children have reached the age of fourteen, they are invited to help out with the younger groups as junior volunteers. Once they reach the age of eighteen, they become adult volunteers. This model provides a constant supply of help from individuals who have benefitted already from attending such groups.

The building is large and inviting. It is decorated with bold colours and has comfy seating. It is a real home from home; a haven for families who have been disadvantaged by the closure of the life force of its community.

Martin and Jackie have clear ideas about how they wish to develop the Exodus Project but the lottery funding which they benefitted from is no longer available. Sadly, they have had to close two of their clubs due to lack of funding. This decision wasn't taken lightly. They do have two charity shops which raises some money and they obtain some funding from outside organisations for the use of their facilities. However, this is clearly not enough to keep their clubs, weekend activities and building going to cater for the ever growing number of children who are benefitting from the work being undertaken here. Neither does it allow for future development.

Exodus do have a Just Giving page which can be found here if you wish to help further their work https://www.justgiving.com/exodus

In addition, you can keep up with activities on their Facebook page here

https://www.facebook.com/search/top/?q=the%20exodus%20project%20barnsley&epa=SEARCH_BOX

www.ingramcontent.com/pod-product-compliance
Lightning Source LLC
Chambersburg PA
CBHW052357220526
45465CB00003BB/1144